BIRTH

BIRTH

A unique visual record – 14 different births

in hospital, at home, caesarian, epidural, breech, twins

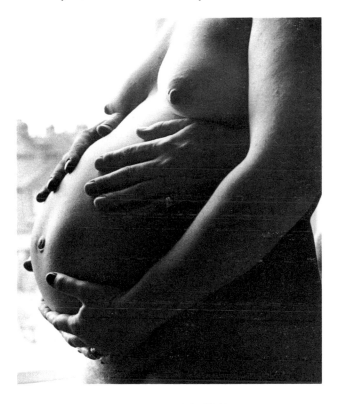

Nancy Durrell McKenna

BLOOMSBURY

First published 1988
Copyright © 1988 Nancy Durrell McKenna
Bloomsbury Publishing Limited,
2 Soho Square, London W1V 5DE

British Library Cataloguing in
Publication Data

Durrell McKenna, Nancy
    Birth.
    1. Childbirth
    I. Title
    618.4

ISBN 0 7475 0177 7

Designed by Marnie Searchwell

Typeset by SX Composing Ltd
Rayleigh, Essex
Printed in Great Britain by BAS Printers,
Stockbridge, Hampshire

Contents

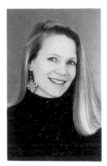

Nancy Durrell McKenna is Canadian, with degrees from McGill and Concordia universities. Since 1976 she has lived in London, working as a freelance photographer.

Her two main interests are development issues in the Third World and pregnancy, birth and child development. She has published with writers Sheila Kitzinger and Miriam Stoppard and is the author of four other books including *Sawubona!* (1982) and *Kwazulu South Africa* (1985). She is married and has two sons.

Foreword

Any woman expecting a baby – especially the first time round – wonders what it is really like to go through childbirth. There is always an element of mystery. It is not just a matter of getting information about practicalities and about the physiology of labour – or even of knowing how much pain there may be. It is more than anything a matter of understanding the often complex emotions of birth – the feelings which are stimulated in all those who participate in it.

In this book Nancy Durrell McKenna, a photographer with a keen eye and a sensitive awareness of these deep feelings, reveals the very heart of the birth experience. She shows how birth was for a group of very different women, their partners, and in some cases their midwives and doctors, too, and lets them speak for themselves. Some had easy births, others very difficult ones. Some labours took a long time, others were very short and sweet.

The result is a vivid and compelling book which is at once realistic, tender and – above all – exciting.

SHEILA KITZINGER

The pain of labour can be bad but it doesn't have to be a bad experience . . .

MIDWIFE

Introduction

The more we know about what happens to our bodies while giving birth the less likely we are to let our fears and anxieties take the experience out of our control. Photographs can and do increase our awareness of what giving birth is like. Photographs fill out the facts and above all dispel much of the anxiety about the birth process.

When I was pregnant I wanted a book which made birth accessible through photographs and stories as told by women and their partners. *Birth* is that book. I have been very privileged to have been part of many births and to have witnessed the complexity of emotions shared by women during this intense event. We experience moments of doubt, fear of losing self control, the monotony of the pain, reactions to our partners and the ultimate realisation that once labour has begun there is no turning back. And we experience moments of humour and great, great joy.

The narrative in *Birth* is based on interviews with the women, their partners and labour staff present at the birth. I was moved by their openness and frankness to tell it as it was . . . and to share with me their experience of birth – an everyday miracle.

Author's acknowledgments
To the women and their partners, thank you. I have learned much and shared with you a very special experience.

I am grateful to the obstetric departments of many hospitals in London and Dublin, in particular to obstetricians Yunus Tayob of the Royal Free Hospital, London, and Dermot MacDonald of the National Maternity Hospital, Dublin, and to general practitioners Jonathan Riddell and Roger Lichy who provided the support for couples to have home births, not to mention the numerous midwives who have shown me the meaning of tender care.

Writing and photographing this book has been all consuming and uplifting. Women rarely give birth between the hours of 9am – 5pm! As one woman in labour said to me, 'It's bad enough having to stay up all night for your own birth, let alone someone else's', but I always returned home on a real high . . . and home is where my support is – my husband Bill and our au pairs, Jose Luis and then Elisa, who were enthusiastic and unflappable. They enabled me to leave without worry when the telephone rang.

Geoff Langan my photographic assistant processed, printed and edited with me. At the end of the day we could still laugh and that says a lot. To good friends Kathryn Berry and Maty Grünberg your artistic input and time was invaluable.

Having an idea about a book and getting it published can seem like worlds apart. I want to thank Kathy Rooney my editor, whose response when I first showed her the proposal was 'that's exactly what I was looking for when I was pregnant', . . . the gap had closed.

Nancy Durrell McKenna

Some men
don't want to see their wives
giving birth because they
wonder what it is going to
do to their sexual
appreciation of them. But
it's part of the same
business, it's a continuation
of making love.

JOHN

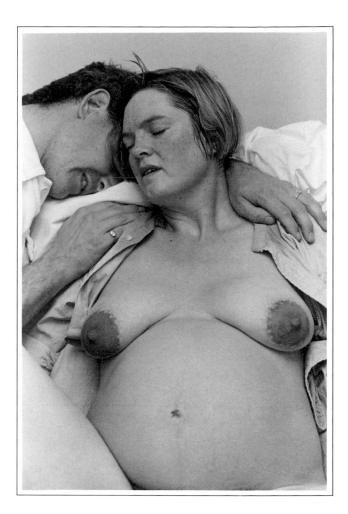

Jennifer and John

Jennifer is thirty-two years old, second
pregnancy. Her first baby came two
weeks early and was delivered after a
very fast labour of four hours. Jennifer
remembers being definitely out of
control and frightened by the speed and
intensity of the contractions. This labour
was six hours.

I am feeling rather worried – I think it's the anticipation of not knowing how long it is going to go on for. I was more scared this time. With Jack, who came two weeks early, I didn't have time to be frightened. When you get to this stage you worry about how this huge lump is going to get out and you realise that it's beyond your control, that nature will take over.

The atmosphere was very cosy in spite of being in a hospital. It felt like we had just rented a room for the night and we had all met there for the birth.

JOHN

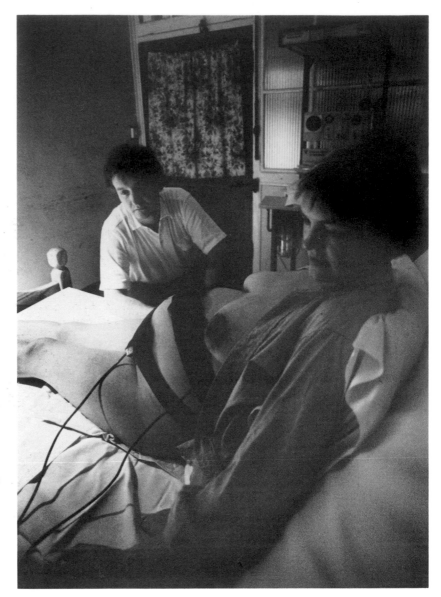

Jenny is being monitored. The top belt monitors the contractions, the bottom belt monitors the foetal heart beat, so we get a read out with two lines. You then compare the foetal heart rate with the contractions to assess how the baby is coping.

MIDWIFE (INGRID)

This was a very peaceful time for me. I was pleased that I only had to keep the foetal heart monitor on for twenty minutes. After that I was monitored intermittently with a portable foetal heart monitor. This allowed me to move around and change positions, whatever felt most comfortable. Just before the baby was born the midwives listened to the baby's heart beat after every contraction.

JENNIFER

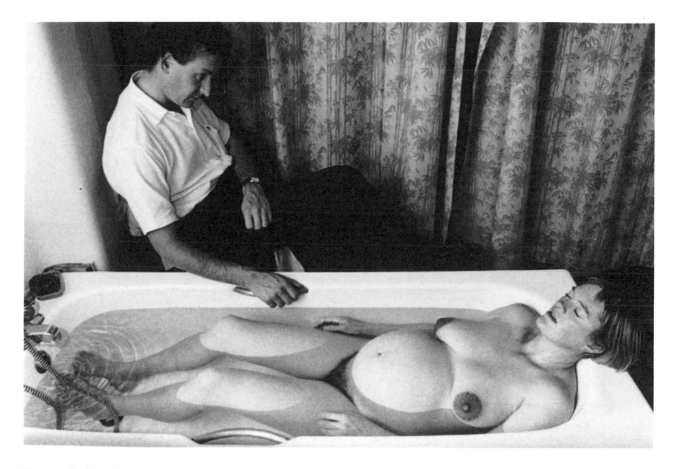

This was before the contractions became unbearable. Jennifer seemed to be anticipating the contractions and enjoying them. She'd smile and say 'That was a tough one', but she seemed to recover quite well between contractions. She was worried about her own performance, about not doing it right.

JOHN

I was able to relax in the bath, and stayed in it about one hour. John was timing the contractions and telling me when I was half way through, which is one of the ways I had been taught to cope with contractions, once you know you are half way through the contraction, the worst is over.

The change from bearable contractions to unbearable started to occur while in the bath and I was considering pain relief.

JENNIFER

Jennifer would grab for the mask quite desperately and that was frightening to watch. It seemed to knock her out for a little bit and then she would remove the mask. Her grip on my hand was very strong.

JOHN

I am a great fan of gas and air. It got me through my first labour, and this one.

JENNIFER

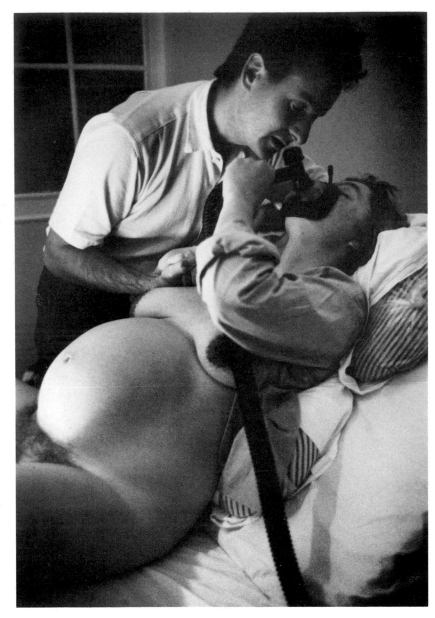

With gas and air, you start breathing it in before you feel the height of the contraction. Ideally, someone is with you, telling you when a contraction is coming – either by timing it or feeling your abdomen. By putting your hand on the abdomen you can feel the contraction building up; when the contraction peaks the abdomen is very hard and it relaxes as the contraction disappears. The gas and air takes you over the height of the contraction. You have to stop breathing it between contractions or you can get dizzy. Gas and air is expelled from the body very quickly and doesn't affect the baby.

MIDWIFE

I suddenly remembered that we had this mineral water spray which would be quite cooling, as well as using the sponge. It's quite fun to have the chance to spray someone in the face and to have them enjoy it. The sponging and spraying was something that I could do that would help.

JOHN

My memory is all a bit hazy but it felt so refreshing, also it was the comfort of knowing that someone was looking after me. I wanted to have John's hand to hold or if John had not been present it would have been one of the midwives.

JENNIFER

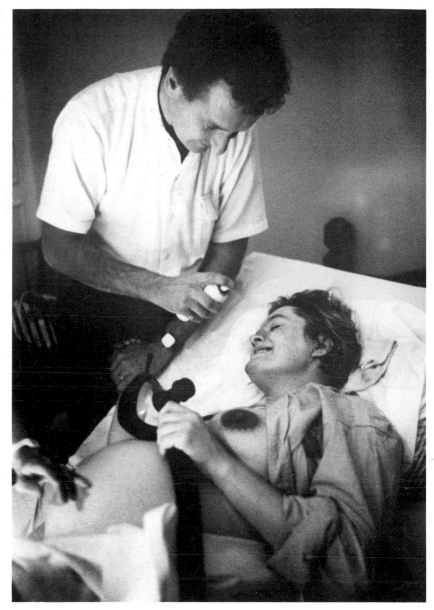

My duty I felt was just to be there, to support and comfort Jennifer, to hold her hand when she was having a bad contraction, to tell her when she was getting to the middle of a contraction, to give her some warning when the next one was coming. It was quite difficult to get close to Jennifer from the side of the bed. It would have been nicer to have been able to sit behind her. I was conscious of only being able to touch her shoulder rather than giving her a hug.

JOHN

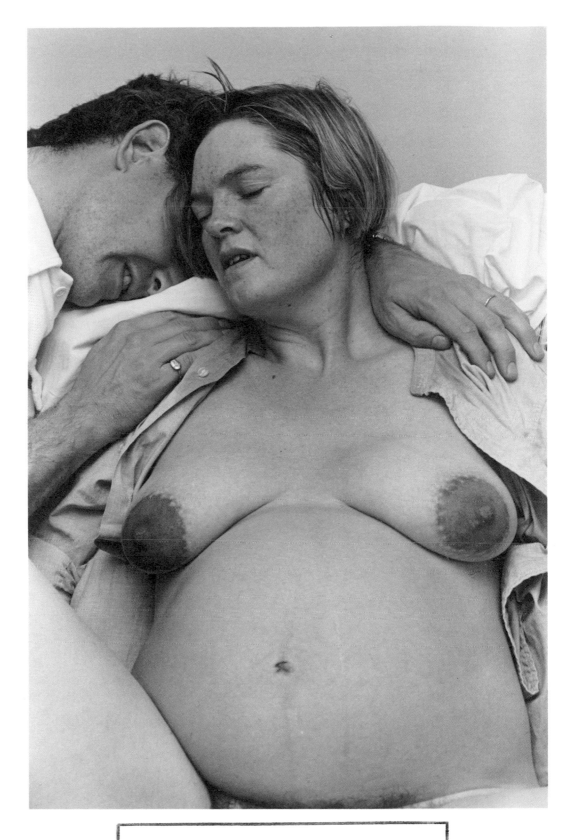

You are the support person, the
someone who is familiar and is
looking after your wife's interests.
When the midwife says pant you can
reinforce that need. You need to be
at the top end supporting, not where
the action is.

JOHN

I remember that feeling of wanting
to push and yet being told that I was
not quite ready. That was very
difficult. It's such an overwhelming
feeling. I was very aware of John
telling me to pant, his familiar voice.

JENNIFER

*The head has just started to appear
(crowning). I am encouraging the head
to flex so that the chin goes on to the
chest. We have established by
abdominal palpation that the baby is
facing Jenny's bottom (occipito
anterior). I am pressing against the
head, you have to use quite a lot of
force to try and flex it down. With
my other hand I am guarding the
perineum, holding it together and
telling Jenny to pant so that when a
contraction comes she doesn't push
uncontrollably and tear the perineum.
(Her perineum did tear a little.) We
don't want to traumatise the tissues
too much – by panting she gently
pushes it out.*

MIDWIFE

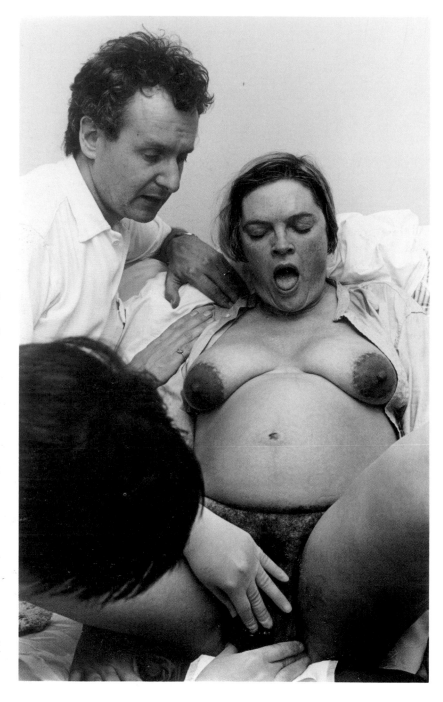

I remember the sensation of tearing
but it wasn't painful – it was a
distant feeling. You imagine that it
would be excruciating but it doesn't
compare with the pain of
contractions.

JENNIFER

18

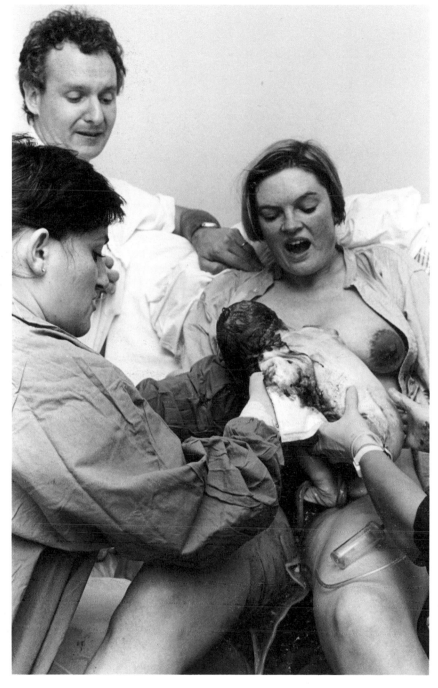

All throughout the pregnancy I did find it difficult to imagine that there was a little person in there. There's not really a baby until the baby is born, then suddenly there he is. Looking at his hands and feet there seemed to be fairly flappy skin as if it was ready for growing into.

JOHN

My hands are around both shoulders, lifting the baby on to Jenny's tummy. The gush of water is the rest of the amniotic fluid. The baby is covered with a fine white mucus called vernix. Once the baby's head and anterior shoulder had been delivered I gave Jenny an injection of syntocinon in her thigh. Syntocinon stimulates the uterus to contract and expels the placenta more quickly than would happen normally. Some women object to syntocinon or any interference with the delivery of the placenta which, under normal circumstances, will come away within half an hour.

MIDWIFE

It was lovely to have the baby come directly on to my chest – with Jack they took him immediately to the ventilator to check him.

JENNIFER

I am clamping the cord in two places.
You must clamp before you cut the
cord otherwise it will bleed. Clamping
is cutting off the blood supply to the
baby. We waited about one minute
before clamping the cord.

MIDWIFE

Some men don't want to see their
wives giving birth because they
wonder what it is going to do to
their sexual appreciation of them.
But it's part of the same business,
it's a continuation of making love.

JOHN

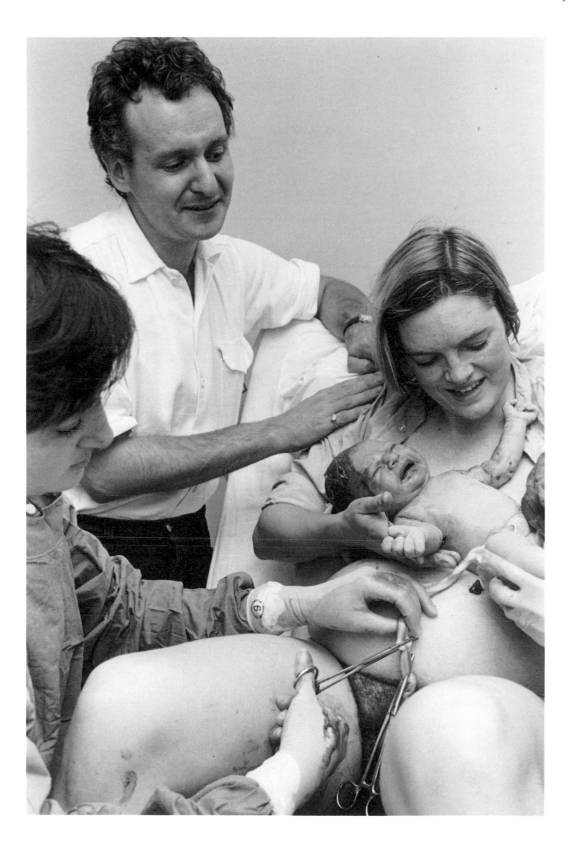

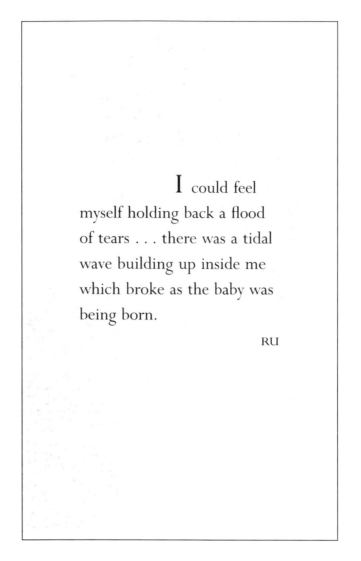

I could feel
myself holding back a flood
of tears . . . there was a tidal
wave building up inside me
which broke as the baby was
being born.

RU

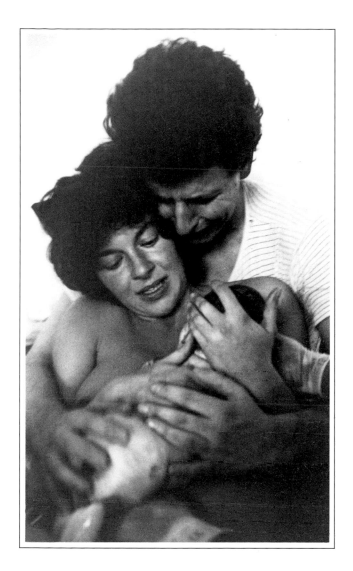

Lesley and Ru

Lesley is twenty-eight years old, first
pregnancy. She delivered at home, after
a sixteen hour labour.

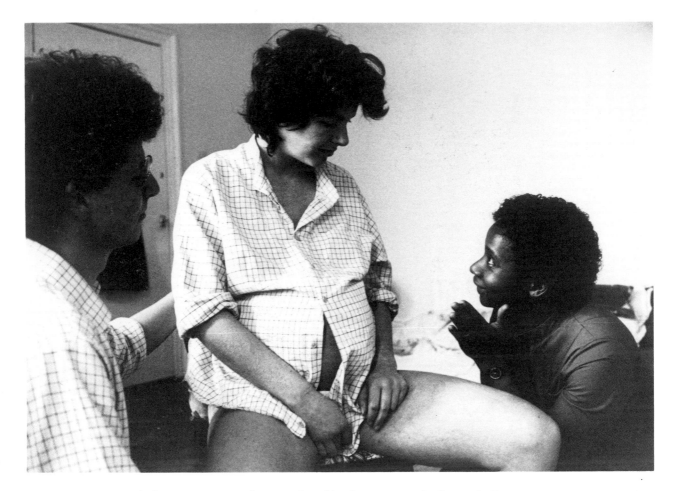

As I was getting out of my car, I could hear Lesley's voice from outside but I thought that she couldn't be fully dilated. I examined her and saw that she was only half dilated, so I said, 'Come on, get yourself together. You are in very early labour, if you start screaming, crying and getting upset now, you've still got the work to do at the end!' So we sat down and had a chat, she had something to drink and eat and was fine. She coped very well with the contractions.

MIDWIFE (JANET)

Janet, my midwife, was brilliant. When she walked into the room, I was coping badly, grunting away like a stuffed pig. She just walked through the door and said, 'Right, that's the end of that noise', got me up off the bed, sorted out my breathing and massaged my neck and lower back. She got me organised without any hassle.

LESLEY

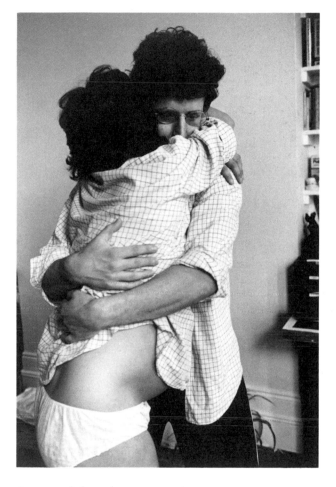

*I suggested that when a contraction
came to stand up and rock from side to
side. Her partner, Ru, took an active
part and from then on it was a very
shared experience.*

MIDWIFE

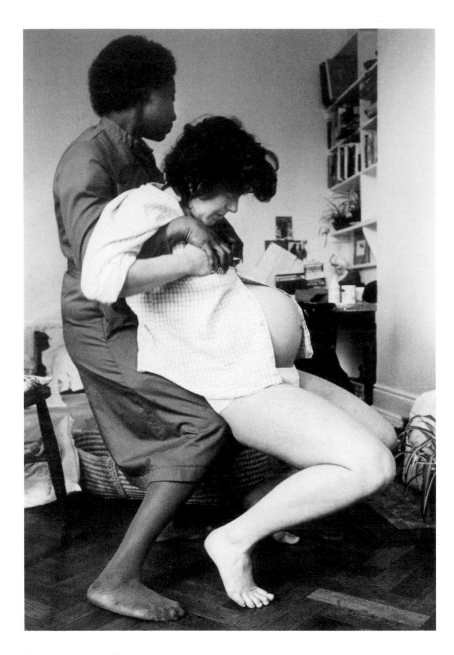

By taking most of Lesley's weight in a supported squat she was able to rock from side to side. I was responding to what she wanted.

MIDWIFE

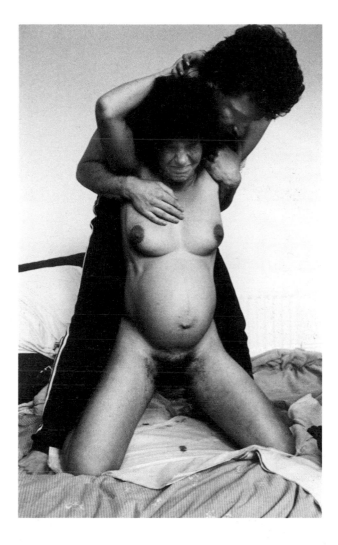

This position felt ace. It must have
been knackering for Ru but it was
just what I wanted – to be able to
hang and bear down with all my
energy to push the baby out.

LESLEY

*Because I was gloved up waiting to do
the delivery, Chris, the GP, listened to
the foetal heart sound. Even when the
head has crowned it is important to
keep listening to the heart sound, until
you can see the baby's face, catch the
blinking or hear a cry, something that
tells you 'I'm alive and well'.*

MIDWIFE

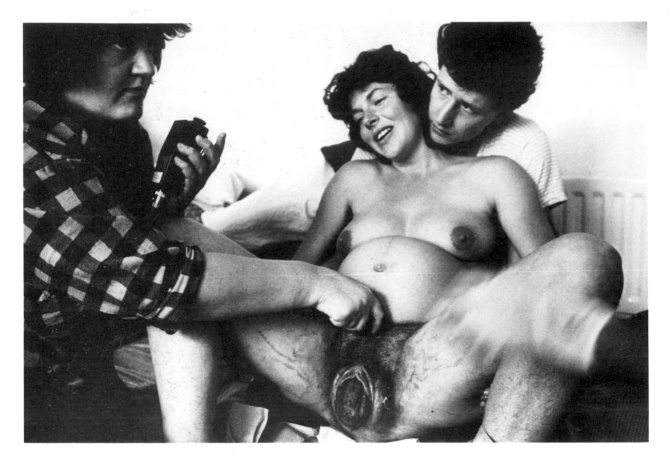

I had expected one hell of a lot of
pain, and the pain definitely was
there, but I was pleased that I didn't
need any pain killers because they
would have interfered too much
with what was going on. I consider
that my pain killers were Janet and
Ru.

LESLEY

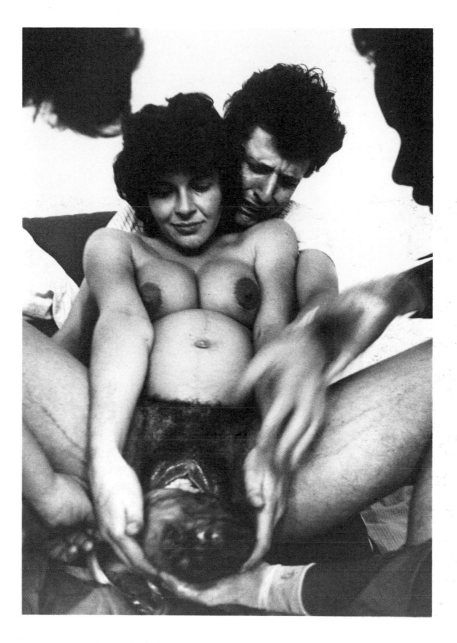

I had checked the cord which was
around the baby's neck, but it was
loose and easily slipped over the head.
Lesley's hands came down to lift the
baby up.

    I took Ru's hands and placed
them on to the baby so that the two
of them brought the baby on to her
tummy.

MIDWIFE

I make it a habit of letting the mother and father bring the baby up on to the mother's tummy so that they can make contact with the baby immediately, even before the legs have been delivered. They have seen the baby for the first time together. Even if the baby's eyes are closed they have made contact with the baby's face.

MIDWIFE

Towards the end of labour, there was a lot of tension building in me. It was a matter of restraining the tears. There had been the nine months and the fact that Lesley had been very late (three weeks) meant that there had been more time for the tensions to grow. Every time Lesley stood on a chair to shut the window I was worried that she might fall. I could feel myself holding back a flood of tears . . . there was a tidal wave building up inside me which broke as the baby was being born. A very liberating experience for me.

RU

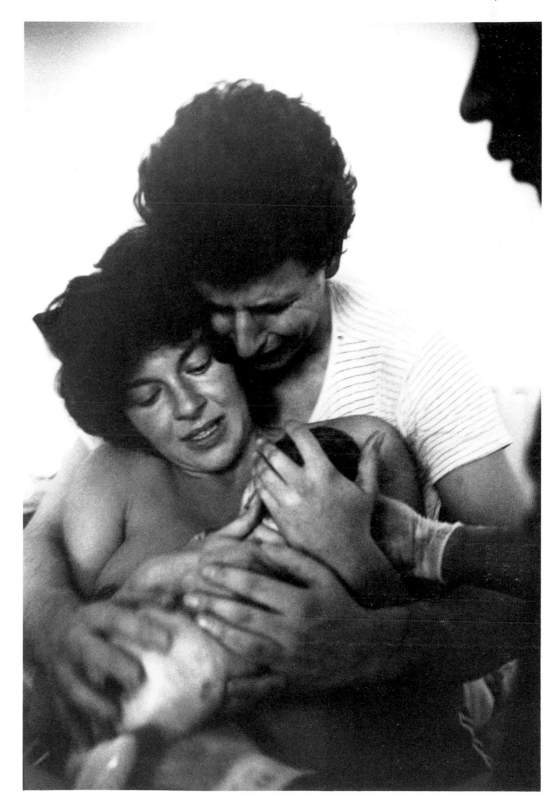

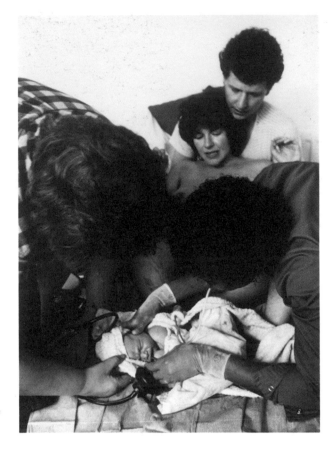

Once the baby had come up on to Lesley's tummy and they had rubbed her, I sucked out the water. What I usually do if the baby is mucousy is to turn her over with the face on the tummy. But this baby had swallowed a lot of water and it was necessary to suck it out. The doctor gave her the oxygen mask to pink her up.

MIDWIFE

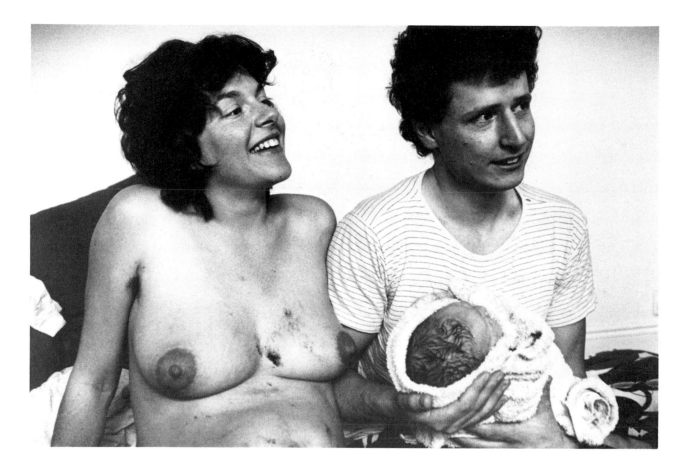

I was away with the fairies and that
lasted three days . . . but the more
interesting thing was that as I was
having my stitches, and Ru was
holding the baby, I found myself
glancing over my left shoulder to
look at this baby that Ru was
holding. It was very uncanny. I was
thinking, that's my baby over there,
and yet I was glad to be a little
distanced from her. It gave me a
break to calm down and to get used
to the idea of this baby being on the
outside of the world. I loved her
because she was my child and
because I had produced her but to
get used to her being there and
to get to know her took time.

LESLEY

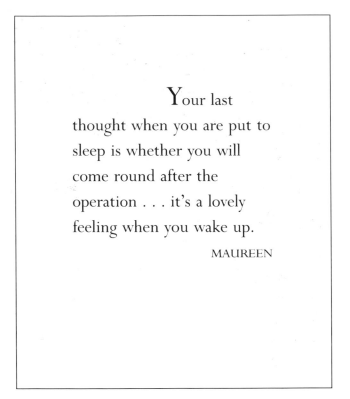

Your last thought when you are put to sleep is whether you will come round after the operation . . . it's a lovely feeling when you wake up.

MAUREEN

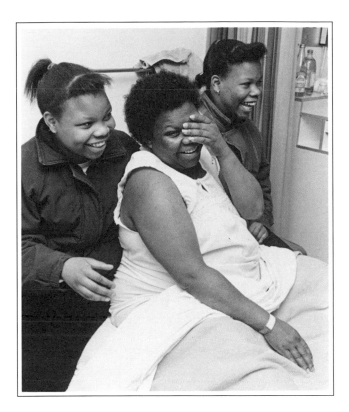

Maureen

Maureen is thirty-six years old, third
pregnancy. Her three babies were
delivered by caesarian section under
general anaesthesia.

My girls Andrea and Samantha are
fifteen and twelve years old. They
were both delivered by caesarian
section under general anaesthesia.
For both pregnancies the pelvic
x-rays had shown that my pelvis was
smaller than the baby's head. This
time I thought about having a
caesarian under epidural anaesthesia
but decided against it on the advice
of medical friends who said I might
feel some sensations, and possibly
pain. The doctors had assured me
that modern anaesthetics are better
now and that I would be awake
within half an hour of having the
baby.

MAUREEN

We are very excited about this baby.
We're sure it's a boy.

ANDREA AND SAMANTHA

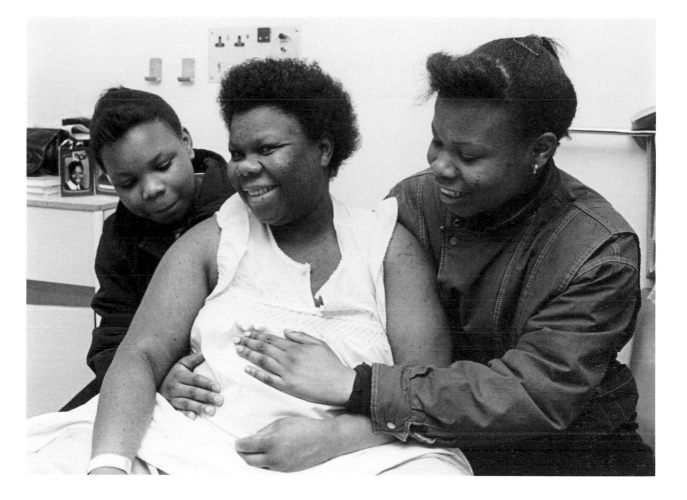

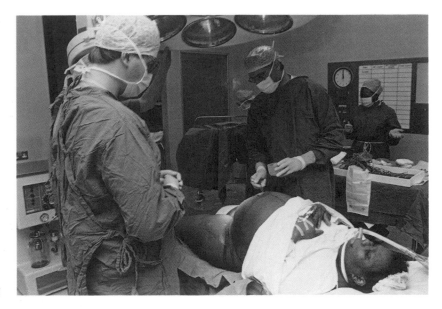

I am cleansing the lower abdomen with antiseptic solution in preparation for making the incision.

OBSTETRICIAN

One must take care that in a caesarian section under general anaesthesia the woman doesn't regurgitate any stomach contents and inhale them. This is one of the most common causes of maternal deaths, although rare. We give the woman oxygen beforehand so that she has a store of oxygen in her lungs and then a rapid induction of anaesthesia intravenously which produces instant sleep. By pressing on the oesophagus below the larynx (the voice box) we block off the stomach from the throat so that no stomach contents can get back, thus reducing the risk of inhalation.

At this stage we put a cuffed tube into her windpipe, the cuff is blown up and that seals off her windpipe so that if anything does come up from the stomach it cannot go down into the lungs. The tube is attached to the ventilator which provides a regular supply of oxygen and removes carbon dioxide. We make sure that she is well oxygenated and very lightly asleep until the baby is born.

ANAESTHETIST

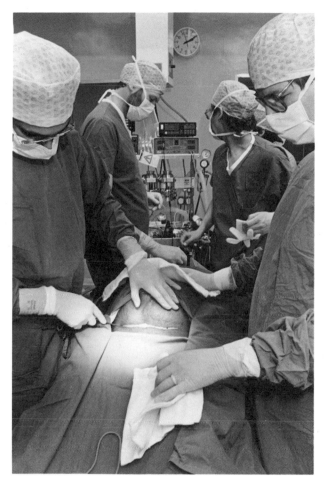

I am making a low transverse incision into the abdomen just above the pubic hair line. Cosmetically it's a very acceptable incision. The pubic hair grows over it so it's probably not visible again. On this occasion there is no blood visible. The blood vessels are deeper lying but you can have small capillary bleeds with this first incision. Between my thumb and index finger you can see scar tissue from her previous caesarians when the incision was done vertically. I have decided not to go through that incision but to choose a new site which is cosmetically nicer, will heal quickly and will allow her to get home sooner. With a history of two previous caesarian sections one would automatically do a third because of the risk of rupture of the uterus at the site of the two previous incisions. This is most likely during labour. The two scars on the uterus no longer have elastic tissue but are composed of fibrous gritty tissue which will not stretch. This weakened area on the uterus may rupture and the rupture pose a risk to both mother and baby. Women who are to have an elective caesarian section come into hospital at thirty-eight weeks. The reason for this early admission to hospital is to exclude the possibility of their going into labour and thus obviating the above risks. Most elective caesarian sections are performed between thirty-eight and thirty-nine weeks of pregnancy.

OBSTETRICIAN

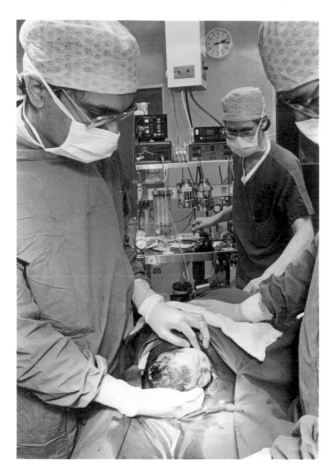

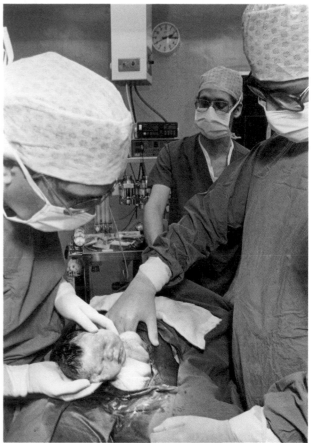

The baby's head is just appearing.
Between the mother's legs which are
covered by a sterile drape you can see
the liquor on the sheets. The liquor is
the fluid which surrounds the baby.

OBSTETRICIAN

My assistant is holding up the upper
part of the abdominal incision while I
deliver the baby's head and shoulders.
It looks as though I am pulling hard
but in fact I am only applying gentle
traction.

OBSTETRICIAN

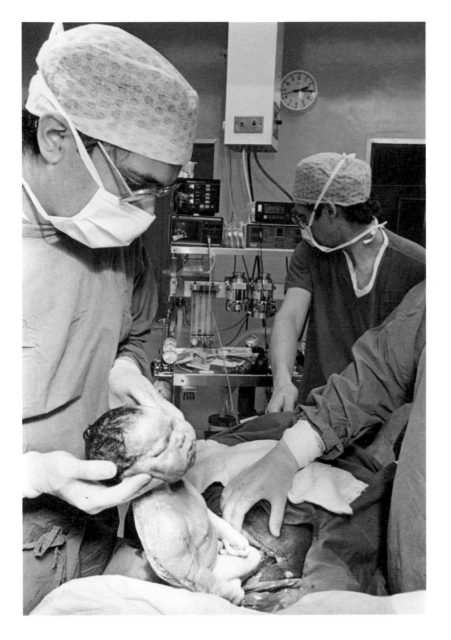

All of the baby is now out. The white
coating which is just visible on the
baby's back is the vernix, the protective
water repellant substance which babies
have.

OBSTETRICIAN

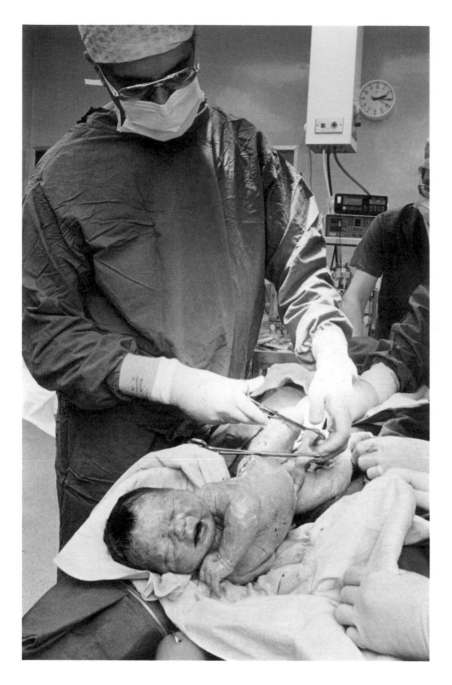

The baby's crying and he's made a face. The cord was felt to stop pulsating. The cord is clamped with very little blood between the clamps.

OBSTETRICIAN

When the cord is being clamped I give the mother syntocinon to make the uterus contract down quickly. At the same time I give a dose of morphine so that she will be comfortable for some hours after she wakes up.

ANAESTHETIST

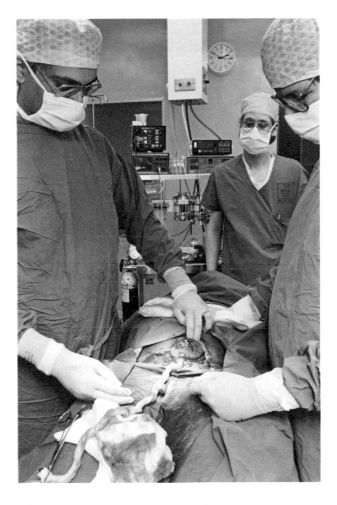

After cutting the cord and handing the baby to the pediatrician, the uterus expells the placenta. Sometimes it's necessary to apply sustained traction on the cord to aid the delivery of the placenta. I am trying to ease the placenta through the opening in the uterus by holding up the upper border of the incision.

OBSTETRICIAN

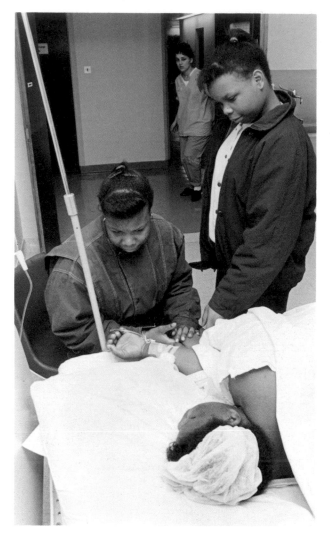

*Modern anaesthetics are metabolised
quite rapidly and therefore the mothers
recover quickly. In the past being able
to hand the baby to the mother after
she had recovered was unusual as she
slept for several hours.*

OBSTETRICIAN

The baby was born at 2.15pm and I
was talking to the girls at 3pm,
although I was a little groggy.

Your last thought when you are
put to sleep is whether you will
come round after the operation . . .
it's a lovely feeling when you wake
up.

MAUREEN

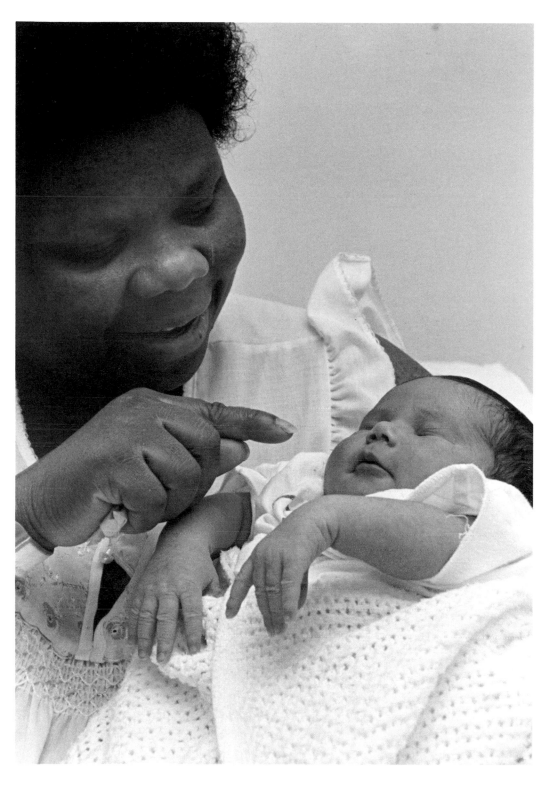

A boy – the girls got what they
wanted. I have a complete family.

I do still wish that it had happened at home. It would have been so much more wonderful, more magical, but you have a baby because you want a child not because you want to give birth.

GENEVIEVE

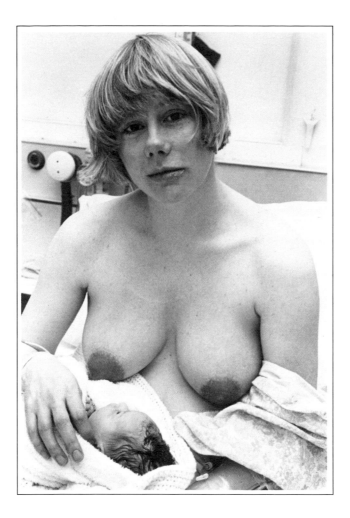

Genevieve and Barry

Genevieve is thirty-two years old, first
pregnancy. She had planned a home
birth but after nineteen hours of labour
was transferred to hospital.

I decided to have a home birth
before I became pregnant. I love my
home and it seemed like the most
natural place for me to give birth.

In some ways the nicest thing
about the labour was being the
centre of attention. Your labour is
the most important thing happening
at that point in time and you are the
only person that everyone is
concentrating on.

GENEVIEVE

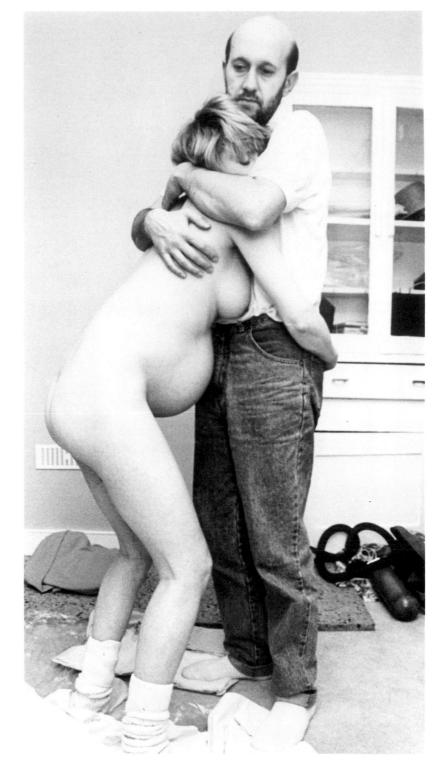

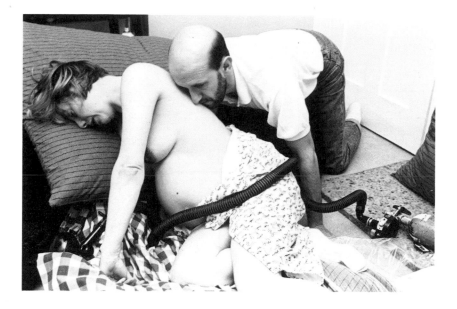

It was good to have Barry so near. I thought that I would communicate a lot with him during the labour but I didn't in the end. I was aware of what was going on around me but I just wanted to turn in on myself and concentrate on what I had to do. I couldn't do that with someone else.

GENEVIEVE

I remember thinking how helpless I felt that I could not really help Genevieve apart from offering comfort and support.

BARRY

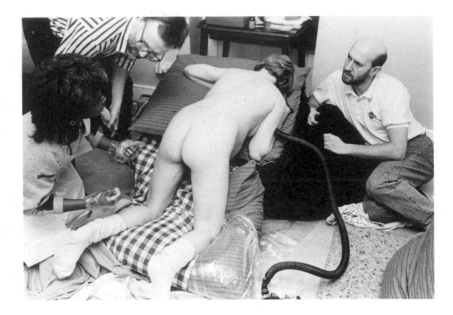

Linda, the midwife, examined Genevieve to find that the cervix had not fully dilated. There was an anterior lip and a rim on both sides of the cervix. I didn't want Genevieve to start pushing yet otherwise the cervix could have become engorged and would have slowed everything up.

The contractions didn't have enough force at that stage to get the baby's head into a better position where it could exert pressure on the cervix to fully dilate it.

GP

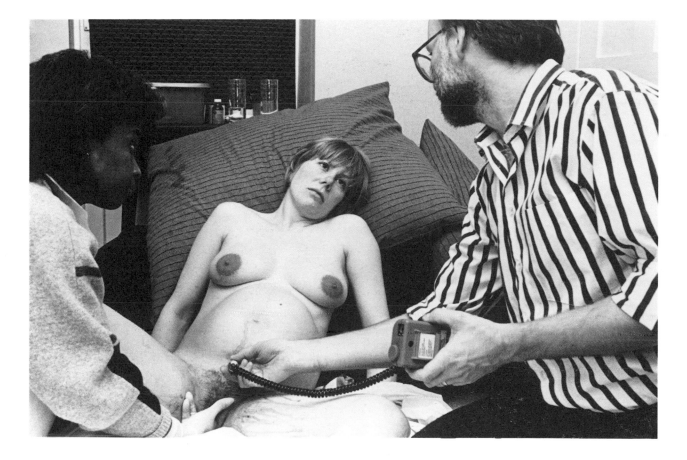

The baby's heartbeat was strong throughout. That in itself was an immense encouragement. To know that inside me was a tiny being waiting to emerge and whose lifeline was still in great working order after all those hours kept my spirits high. However, when contractions slowed down from one every two minutes at 11.30pm to one every five minutes at 1.30am. I felt depressed and dejected. I had a pessimistic feeling after that that things weren't going to go as I had wanted them to.

GENEVIEVE

With the cervix 9cm dilated Genevieve should have been at the extreme end of labour, with contractions coming every two to three minutes. But it wasn't like that, it was very calm. The intensity that should have come just before the pushing was nowhere near.

GP

It had been a long labour, Genevieve was tired and we didn't think she had the reserve of energy. We made the decision to go to hospital to give help with the contractions.

Two hours before Genevieve was transferred to hospital we knew it was inevitable. Often we just have to work through that time, providing the baby is safe, before the woman and family really feel too that the time has come to go into hospital, otherwise they may feel that they have been dragged from the home.

GP

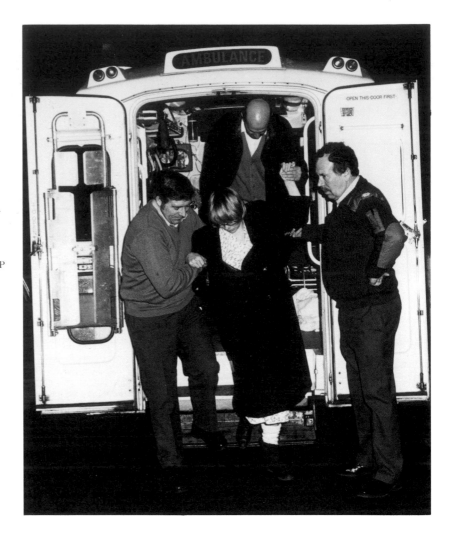

When the decision was taken to go into hospital events progressed quickly and smoothly. I let Barry pack my bag, only to discover later in hospital that the essentials like underwear had been omitted but a facial mask had been included.

Within ten minutes of the ambulance arriving we were in our first room at the hospital. The atmosphere felt good – low lights, dark floor and a birthing bed – but the contractions did not progress. I had to move to an adjacent room where the equipment for induction and monitoring was readily accessible. What had been low tech until then progressed fairly rapidly to high tech.

GENEVIEVE

A syntocinon drip was set up and a scalp electrode applied to the baby's head. When the uterus is stimulated to produce extra contractions an accurate measurement of the baby's heart beat must be recorded.

GP

I was worried now about Genevieve and the baby . . . the air of tranquility and confidence from the staff reassuring me that everything would be okay was a great relief . . . but the midwife did have her own way of doing things. I remember her saying 'I want you to have this baby on your side'.

BARRY

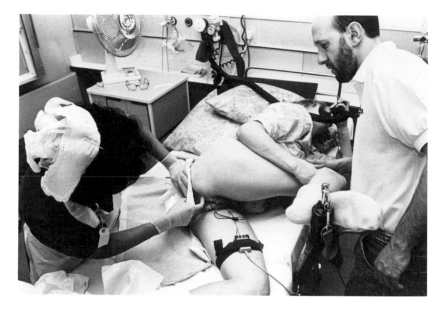

Throughout the labour at home I had tried many different positions to find a comfortable way of dealing with contractions. I always came back to being on all fours and assumed that I would give birth in this position.

With the syntocinon drip the contractions felt so strong that when the midwife suggested that I lie on my side I did it. I thought that regardless of the position that I was in the baby would come anyway. I couldn't see the advantage of getting on all fours at that point.

Gas and air was a great help at this stage. I was glad that I had learned how to use it properly during the early stages of labour at home.

GENEVIEVE

53

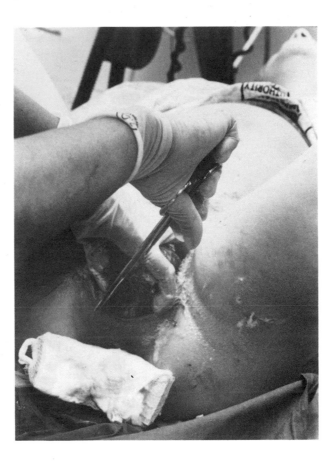

Pushing was very hard and
frustrating. I imagined that when I
started pushing the baby would
come quite quickly but she just kept
slipping back. I had that feeling that
with one extra push the head would
come out but then the contraction
would fade away and the head would
slip back. I needed two small
episiotomies.

GENEVIEVE

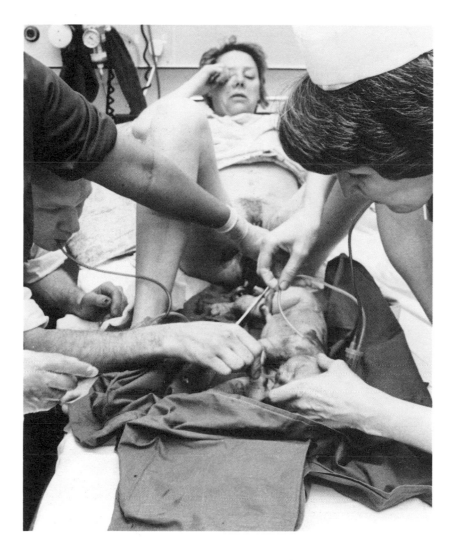

*The pediatrician and midwife sucked
out the baby's nostrils and mouth
before the baby had been completely
delivered in the hope that with the first
cry not much meconium and secretions
would be inhaled.*

GP

I had felt every part of her body –
the head, shoulders, knees and feet.
She just slithered out with all this
warm gushing water. It was the most
wonderful feeling in the world.

GENEVIEVE

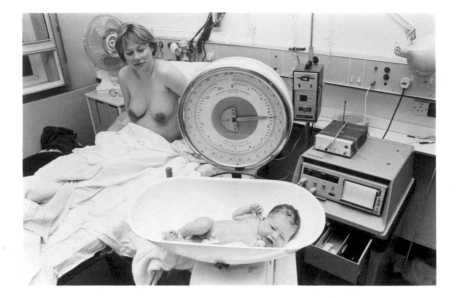

I was very disappointed when she wasn't given to me immediately. I caught a glimpse of her as they rushed her to the other side of the room to check her over. She looked grey and slimy but I knew that she was okay. During the pushing meconium had appeared in the liquor and the pediatrician was called in. The meconium may have been due to stress on the baby.

Once I had seen her I knew that I would never mistake another baby for mine as I had often heard other mothers say they were frightened of doing.

When they brought her to me about ten minutes later she had already been cleaned and wrapped. I had so much wanted to see and hold her in the state she was in at birth just as I had wanted to examine the placenta but I only saw it as it was being delivered. I did look closely at the cord and was amazed that it was so thick – I had imagined it to be thin and stringy.

I just can't help feeling that if I had tried harder I could have done it on my own.

I do still wish that it had happened at home. It would have been so much more wonderful, more magical, but you have a baby because you want a child not because you want to give birth.

GENEVIEVE

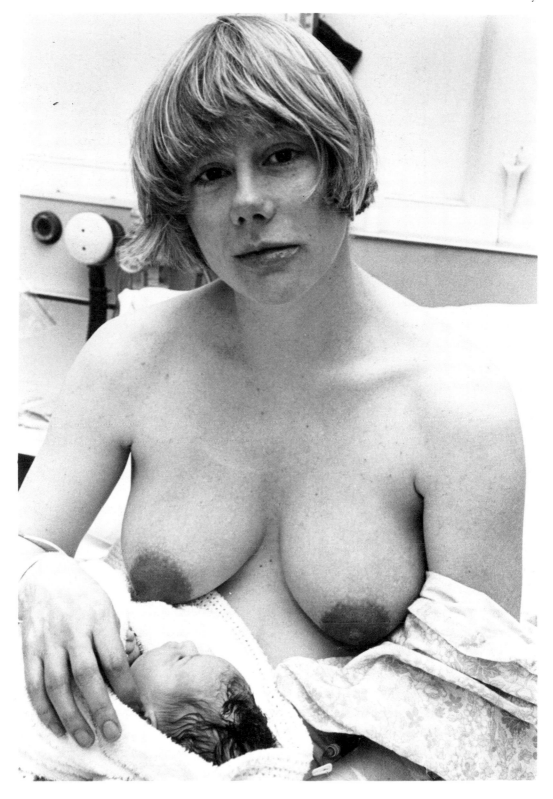

I felt such a
relief to have him born. I lay
back and thought whew it's
over . . . and then I felt a
kick . . .

CLAIRE

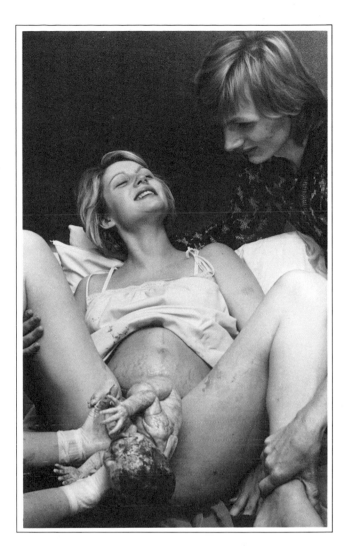

Claire
and Dave

Claire is nineteen years old, first
pregnancy. At forty-one weeks labour
was induced and she gave birth to twins.

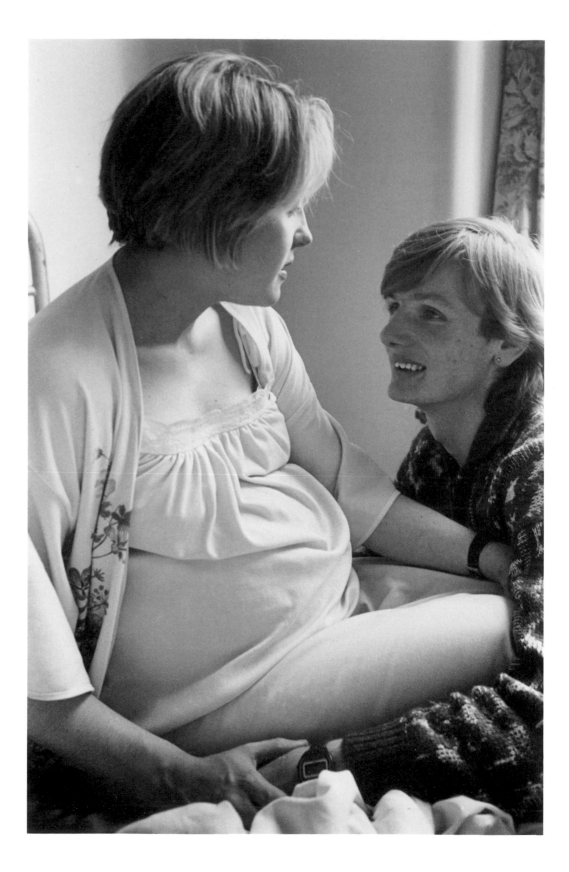

I became pregnant while on the pill. (I had had an ear infection and had been on antibiotics which had upset the cycle.) I discovered that I was pregnant at about ten weeks. Shortly afterwards I was admitted to hospital as I had become dehydrated because I couldn't hold down any food or fluids. Between eight to fourteen weeks I was very sick and during weeks fourteen to sixteen I felt queasy but afterwards I felt just grand. A scan showed that I was carrying twins. It was a big shock – I was horrified at the thought. I hadn't got used to the idea of being pregnant, let alone having twins. I never really got used to the idea of having twins until they were born. Dave, my boyfriend, was shocked as well but consoled me. My mother was great about it which helped a lot.

At forty-one weeks I was induced in the morning by having my membranes broken. It was quite painful but once it was over I felt fine. Dave and I spent the rest of the day waiting and praying for the labour to start. Dave was excited and looking forward to it. Early evening, while I was eating, I started getting terrible cramps and thought that it was due to something I had eaten. When I couldn't go to the toilet I realised that I must be in labour. I vomited. Sister examined me and said that I was 1cm dilated. Labour had finally begun at 6.30pm.

CLAIRE

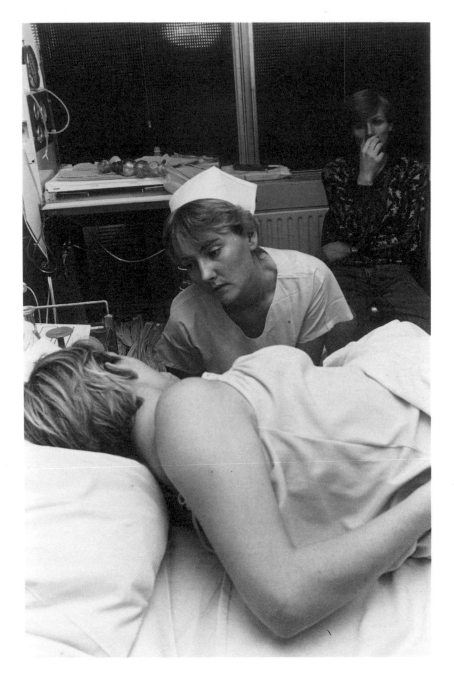

I wouldn't have made it without the midwife – she was terribly nice and kept me calm – there were times when I really felt like screaming.

CLAIRE

The eye to eye contact is so important between midwife and woman. Claire was so attentive. When she was having a contraction she did quiet rhythmic breathing.

MIDWIFE

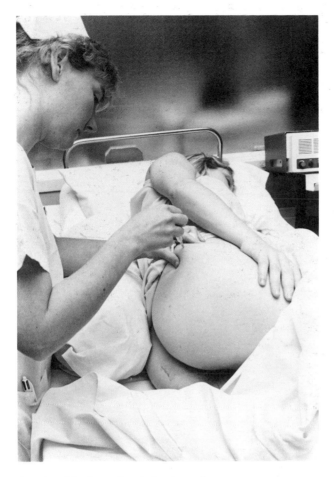

At 11pm I had my first injection of
pethidine, and the second at 1.45am.
The pethidine made me feel very
drowsy but it didn't help the pain. I
felt drugged and it was hard for me
to function. I wasn't aware of what
was going on. I would have liked to
have been more awake and alert in
the early part of labour.

CLAIRE

*50mg of pethidine, gives some pain
relief and helps relax. It usually lasts
about two hours.*

MIDWIFE

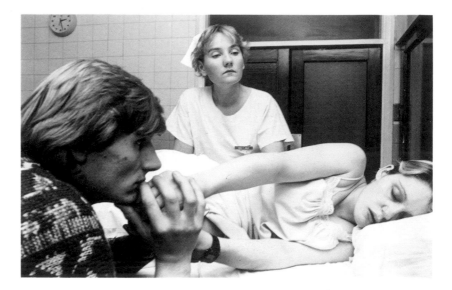

Dave was worried and knackered, he never thought that it would last as long as it did – twelve hours. He thought that it would be over in a couple of hours. Whenever I asked him how he was feeling he always repeated, 'I just want it to be over'.

He annoyed me at first because he tried to chat and I didn't want to talk. I was thinking of sending him out. When he was rubbing my back he was half killing me, but when he was just sitting there it was fine. I was glad that he was there, but I didn't want him hassling me.

I remember wanting to hold the midwife's hand. If she moved away I wanted to hold something – Dave's head – I didn't want to be left alone.

I had constant back pain, it felt like the bottom of my spine was splitting in half all the time – such terrible pressure.

I was going to ask the midwife just to knock me out, section me and get it all over with but then I kept thinking of all the other women who have had babies and I thought if they can do it then I can.

CLAIRE

Rubbing my hand along the sacral part of Claire's back helped to relieve some of the pain. I observed the foetal heart monitor, assessing the length, strength and frequency of the contractions.

MIDWIFE

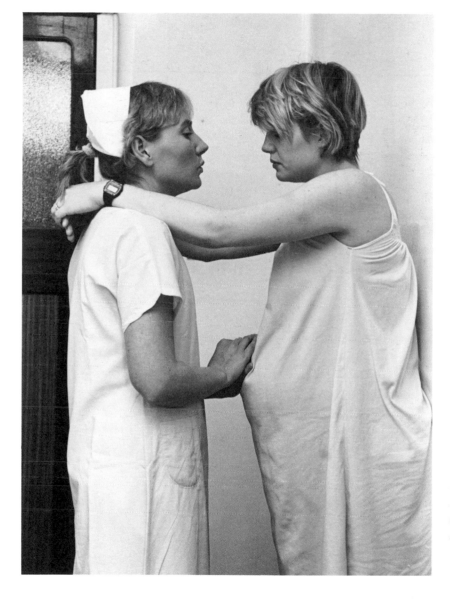

I didn't believe that if I got up and walked around that it would speed labour along. At first I wasn't willing to try. I was too tired. I could hear Dave and the others suggesting that I get up but I thought, 'Oh I wish they would leave me alone, they don't know what they're talking about!'. It was the thought of moving off that high bed which was so daunting. But once I got up and walked around I felt grand.

Gentle pressing on my tummy felt good and relieved some of the pressure of a contraction. In ante-natal classes we had been told to fix our eyes on an object but I couldn't find anything suitable to focus on. It was a great help to keep my eyes open and to have eye contact with Geraldine my midwife.

CLAIRE

I encouraged Claire to try walking and to keep mobile. Keeping mobile tends to shorten the length of labour and takes a woman's mind off the pain and the endurance of labour. By pressing my hand lightly on Claire's abdomen I could feel the contractions of the uterus, and in this way assess whether Claire was having sufficient uterine action.

MIDWIFE

The foetal scalp electrode is linked up to the foetal heart monitor. It monitors the foetal heart continuously but it can be disconnected for the woman to walk around or go to the toilet.

MIDWIFE

I dreaded it when the midwife said that she was going to clip a scalp electrode on to the baby's head but I didn't feel any pain. It was only annoying to have to have the straps undone each time that I wanted to get up and move around. I found it agony to lie on my back.

CLAIRE

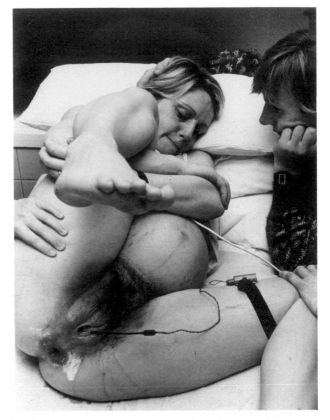

When Claire had the urge to push I examined her to make sure that her cervix was fully dilated. The pouting anus and stretching perineum are good signs that the baby's head is far down. With the first stages of pushing lying on one side can help the baby's head to rotate and get around the part of the sacrum. But in Claire's case, carrying twins, as with those women whose bump is large, it is not a comfortable method of pushing.

MIDWIFE

I found this position very uncomfortable. There was too much to think about co-ordinating: put your head on your chest, hold your breath, pull your leg up and push all at the same time. Pushing was more difficult than I had anticipated. I felt such a strain on my eyes and heart.

CLAIRE

Claire pushed very well all the time, lips closed getting maximum effort out of each push.

MIDWIFE

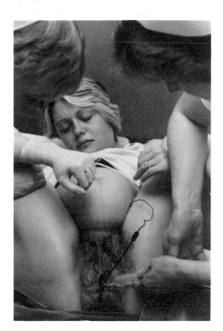 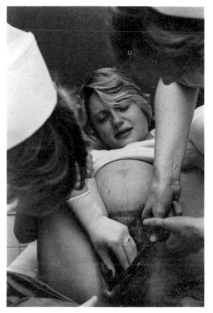

I injected a local anaesthetic into the muscles and tissues of the perineum to numb it in preparation for an episiotomy.

With the previous push, there had been a little trickle of blood coming over the perineum. I felt that it was better to do an episiotomy and have it repaired properly than to have to repair later what could have been very painful vaginal or labial lacerations. Episiotomies are not done routinely with twins. What weighed my decision in this instance was that I couldn't be sure whether the second baby was coming head first, and if it was breech it would have been important that there was an episiotomy, to facilitate the delivery.

STAFF MIDWIFE

By placing my hand on the top of the baby's head I am preventing the baby from coming out too quickly when the episiotomy is being performed. This also ensures that the episiotomy is not further extended.

MIDWIFE

When they did the episiotomy I felt a sensation rather than pain.

CLAIRE

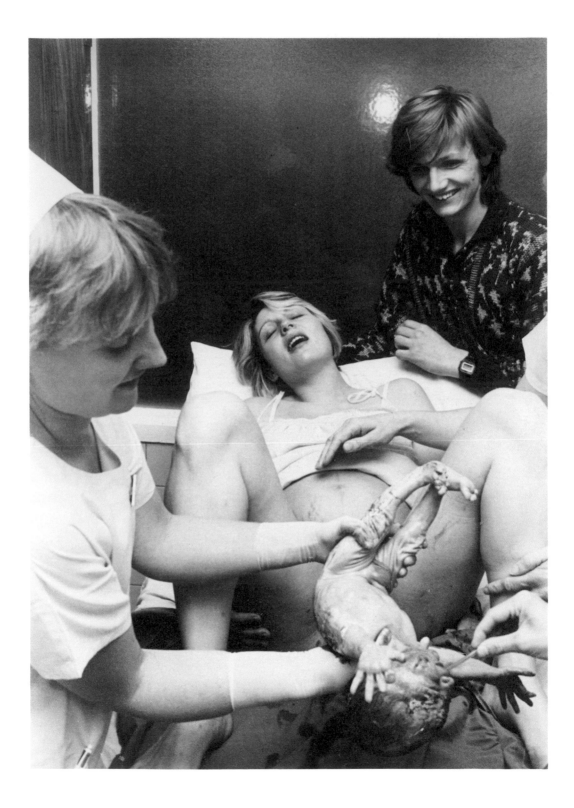

The baby was delivered upside down to aid drainage of any secretions inhaled. The pediatrician cleared the baby's airways by sucking the mucus from the mouth and nose with an extractor. A pediatrician is always present at the delivery of twins, as one can never be sure of the condition of the second.

MIDWIFE

I felt such a relief to have him born. I lay back and thought whew it's over . . . and then I felt a kick . . . I was so nervous holding him, he was so slippery – I was afraid to really look at him in case there was something wrong, but when I saw that he was so perfect I was grateful.

CLAIRE

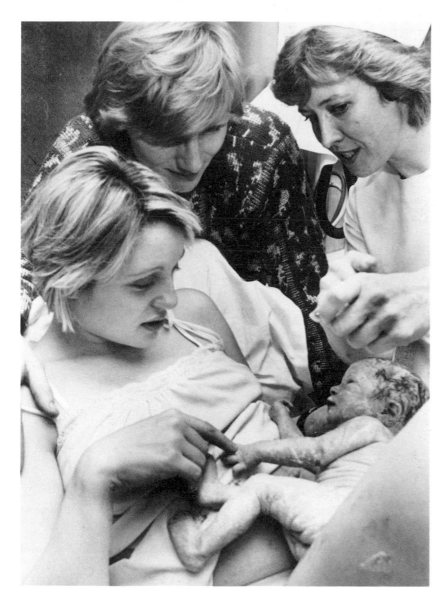

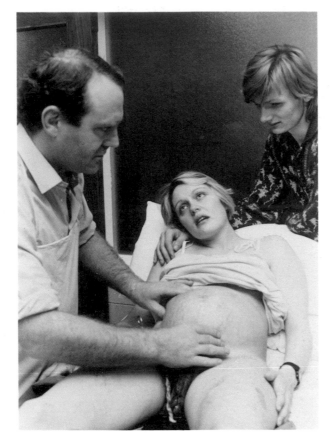

I palpated Claire's abdomen and found that the second baby was lying transversely. The baby's bottom was up to the right and the baby's head was towards the mother's left thigh. Externally, while the midwife held the baby's bottom in position I rotated the head clockwise so that the head was down and ready to be delivered.

OBSTETRICIAN

I was nervous. I didn't know what to expect. I felt pressure as the baby was moving but it was not painful.

CLAIRE

Then I examined Claire internally to confirm that yes, I had turned the baby to head and secondly to confirm that it was head only, and that there was no hand or foot presenting with the head. I ruptured the membranes with amniotomy forceps, after which Claire began pushing and had a spontaneous delivery.

There is no set limit between delivery of twins. Most people would consider that the second twin should be delivered within thirty minutes of the first baby but provided that the mother and second baby are in good condition following delivery of the first one wouldn't try and rush anything.

OBSTETRICIAN

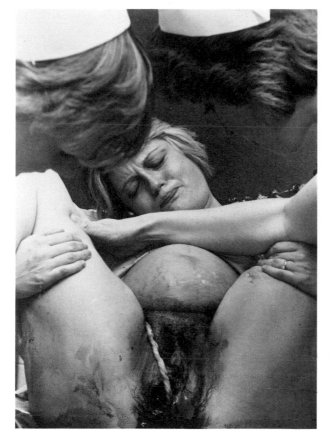

It was very sobering to think that I had to do it all over again. I thought that it would be the same procedure as with the first and that I'd die before I got the second one out but it only took one good push and I knew the head was there and that it would be quicker this time, although the strain was the same.

Pushing them out wasn't difficult, it's just I was so tired I didn't think I had any energy left . . .

CLAIRE

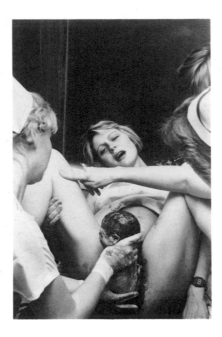

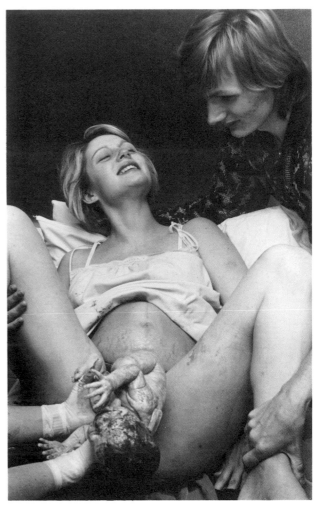

I felt even more relief when the
second baby came out because I
knew then that it was finally over.

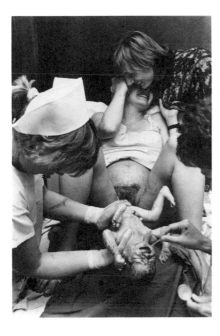 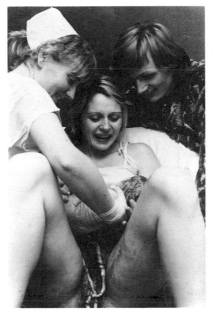 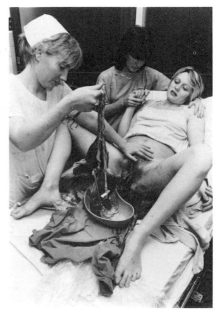

Dave just kept saying, 'It's a girl. It's a girl', and convincing me that it was.

I never thought that we would have a boy and a girl. It was too much to hope for. I thought it would be two girls and Dave thought two boys. When we saw our girl we were so chuffed.

CLAIRE

I delivered the placentae by controlled cord traction. With twins we distinguish between the two placentae by putting two clamps on the umbilical cord of the second placenta. In the event that any abnormalities were noted in one of the placentae it would be important to know which twin it belonged to.

MIDWIFE

I had always thought that the placenta just slipped away and you didn't notice it but I did.

CLAIRE

When I was in labour I thought I'm never going to do this again. It's awful, I don't know how any woman does it twice, they're fools but two hours after the birth, it didn't seem so bad and five days later I thought there was nothing to it and could easily do it again . . .

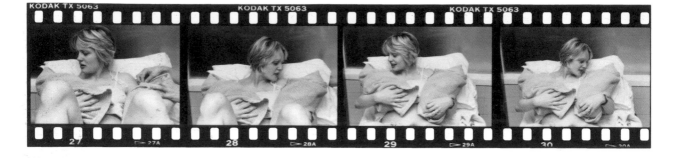

Giving birth was the easiest part, it's afterwards when you bring them home that it dawns on you. For a while I felt as if I wasn't living in the real world. It was hard to adjust to them, hard to believe that they were mine. I didn't feel responsible for them at first because I didn't feel that there was any bond between us but I do now. The bonding has just come on me gradually. They are mine to look after, and I love them but it's frightening as well.

CLAIRE

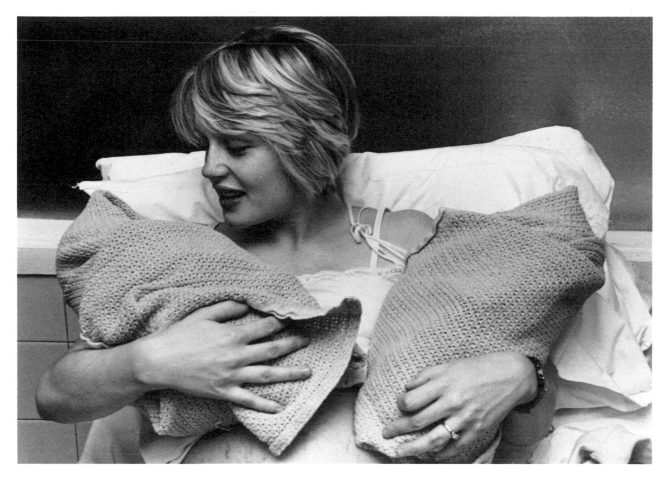

Sean born at 6.45am 5lb 7oz.   Charlene born at 7.00am 5lb 9oz.

I waited seven years before having a second child. I was still frightened by the post operative difficulties I had had after Chi's birth and worried about whether I could cope with two children.

DONNA

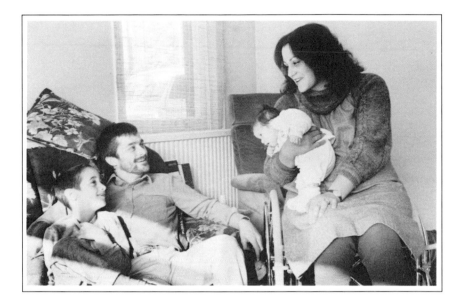

Donna

Donna is thirty-one years old and has been disabled since the age of fifteen. This is her second pregnancy. Both babies were delivered by caesarian section under general anaesthesia.

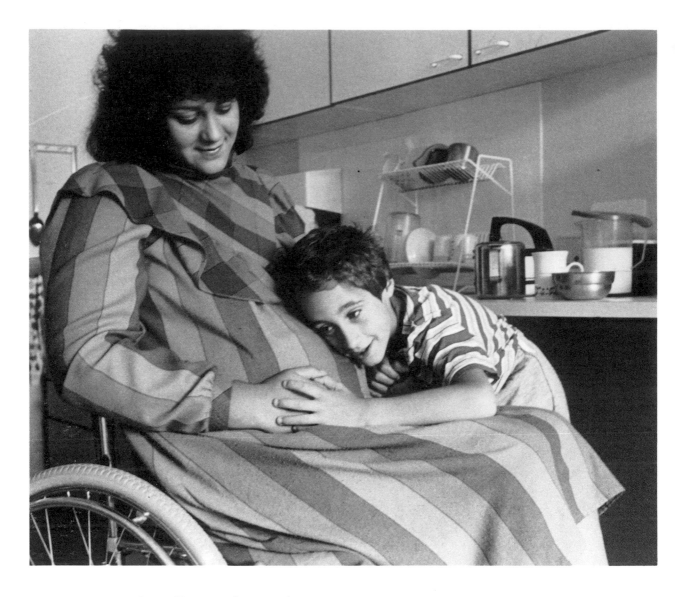

I am a T6 incomplete paraplegic
woman paralysed from under the
bust down. My disability is due to a
spinal abcess I had when I was
fifteen years old. The 'incomplete'
means that I have some feeling,
although I have no surface feeling. I
can't feel slight touch, but I can feel
inner pains.

When I was twenty-four, my first son, Chi, was born. Throughout my pregnancy, I was told that I should have a normal vaginal delivery without complications. During the labour I was able to feel the contractions although not to the same extent as an able bodied woman would have. I was monitored throughout. Paralysed women with damage in the high thoracic or cervical regions of the spinal cord will feel their labour pains in their heads. There's a pressure on the back of the neck and a feeling as if you are going to pop. These headaches result from a dramatic rise in blood pressure caused by uterine stimulation with each contraction. The raised blood pressure must be controlled to avoid possible brain damage.

After being in labour for twenty-four hours with my first baby my cervix had not dilated past 3-4cm, the baby was showing signs of distress so a caesarian was performed. My husband, Tim, was with me during labour but not present during the operation. I was very unhappy about having a caesarian as I was not mentally prepared for it. I remember feeling very cheated afterwards listening to the women in the post natal ward talking about their labours. Chi was born at midnight. He was then taken to the special care baby unit to be checked over but I didn't see him until lunchtime and felt that I had missed out on that early bonding with him.

I waited seven years before having a second child. I was still frightened by the post operative difficulties I had had after Chi's birth and worried about whether I could cope with two children.

After Chi's birth I had a lot of problems with my bladder. This is one of the complications for disabled women having a caesarian – extra care must be taken with the handling of the bladder, bowel and kidneys.

My bladder seized up five times which means that I couldn't pass urine and therefore had to be catheterised each time. I breastfed Chi during those returns to hospital but found that because I was unwell the milk started drying up.

Moving in or out of bed, going from bath to toilet to chair involves lifting myself with my arms. Every time I lifted myself I pulled on my stitches. Happily, I have a good healing skin so no permanent damage was done.

Paraplegic women who deliver vaginally often do so quite effortlessly. Because they do not feel the full impact of the contractions they are not so tense and allow the natural rhythm of the contractions to push the baby out. Should stitches be necessary due to tearing or an episiotomy, extra care must be taken not to sit on them directly. This can be difficult for the paraplegic woman who relies on her wheel chair, so it's best to stay in bed until the stitches have healed. The post natal care is a strong argument for a paraplegic

woman to choose a hospital with a spinal unit. These hospitals are aware of the problems and are equipped to deal with the needs of the disabled woman. Stoke Mandeville hospital, where I chose to go, like to bring the pregnant women in two weeks before their due date. During this period they monitor the well-being of both mother and baby and assess when she is ready to go to the labour ward of the general hospital – a paraplegic woman may not necessarily be able to feel when she is in labour. Before both my labours I slept for most of the preceding twenty-four hours, an indication for me that labour would soon begin. Post natally once the gynaecologist and obstetrician were confident that all was well with me and my baby I returned to Stoke Mandeville hospital where they cared for my 'spinal' side.

DONNA

I was still hopeful of having a vaginal delivery with my second baby but the labour progressed in a similar fashion to that of the first. After thirty-six hours of labour my cervix had not dilated past 3.5cm. However, this time a spinal injuries sister, who I am very close to, was with me during my caesarian operation. She became 'the conscious me, my eyes' and later recounted the proceedings to me in vivid detail. She knew my anxieties about having an operation and she knew how sad I was not to have seen Chi until several hours after he was born. She held Simeon, my second son, moments after he was born, and brought him to me as soon as I had been stitched up. I was still quite hazy but I remember very well holding him . . . important for me. That close bond continues between us.

DONNA

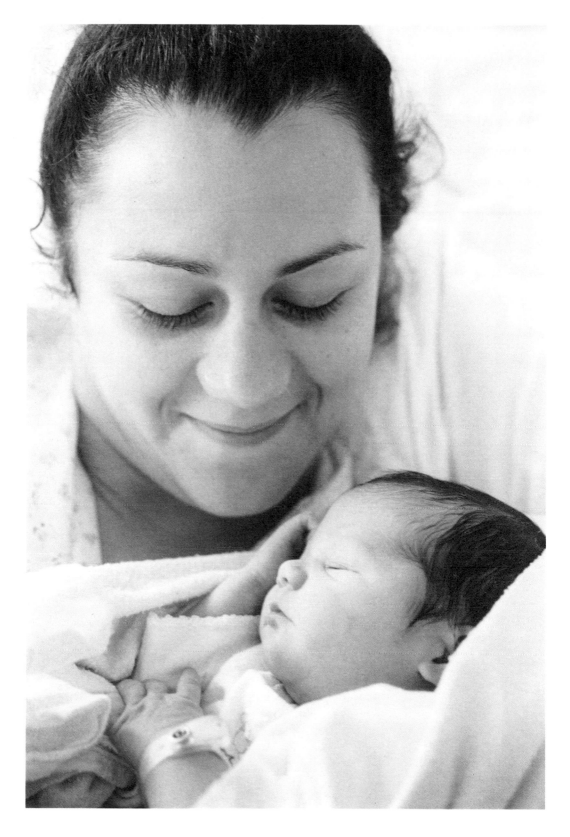

I remember
someone saying, 'It's a boy'
and hearing an awful lot of
crying. I didn't realise he was
out until he was appearing
by my left shoulder. I was
totally stunned and Ken
burst into tears.

LESLEY

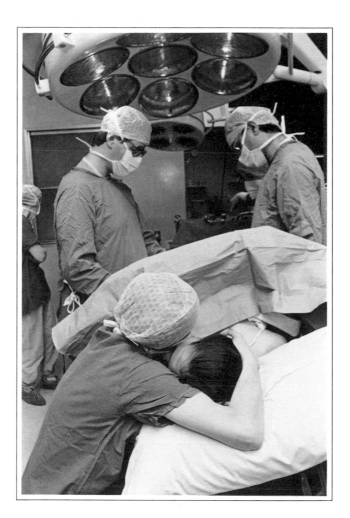

Lesley and Ken

Lesley is twenty-three years old. Last year she had a miscarriage at ten weeks. Lesley had an elective caesarian section under epidural anaesthesia for a breech baby.

During the thirty-eighth week of my pregnancy, the baby became breech. I had had such a fantastic pregnancy, blooming all the way. The breech came as a shock to me – for it all to go wrong at the end seemed like the end of the world. I was very upset.

The pelvic x-ray indicated that my pelvis was slightly small and the baby was bigger than average. It was touch and go whether I could have a normal delivery. The odds favoured a caesarian. I felt that rather than risk going through labour and at the end of the day have to have an emergency caesarian because the baby was stuck, I would rather have a caesarian that was planned from the start. I was influenced by what the doctors had said.

Until the day of the operation I hadn't decided whether to have an epidural or a general anaesthetic. I swayed towards the general – I thought that it would be much easier to go to sleep, and when I woke up it would all be done. But I thought that afterwards I would feel that I had missed out.

Initially, my husband Ken wanted me to have an epidural because he wanted to be with me and therefore me to be awake. However once I was admitted to hospital he got cold feet and said that perhaps he shouldn't be there as he might pass out, make a fool of himself and not be of any use to me. He was worried about what he would see. I felt then that if Ken didn't want to be there I would have a general anaesthetic. Early morning on the day of the operation Ken told me that he wanted to be with me and I had already decided to have an epidural anaesthetic. I'm very glad that I did.

LESLEY

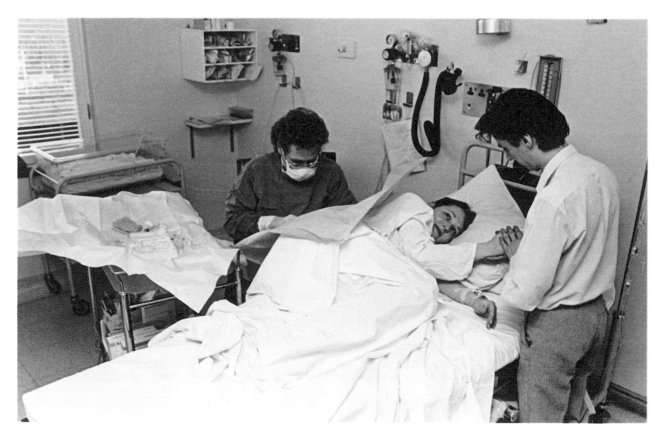

It was very painful when the first local anaesthetic was put in but apart from an electric shock sensation going down my legs I didn't feel anything. I was anxious about what it would be like and surprised that there was little pain. I would recommend an epidural.

At first my abdomen and the small of my back felt very heavy and then my legs went very hot and numb. Because my ribcage was numb I had a very strange sensation when I tried to take a deep breath – as if it wasn't working.

LESLEY

As more literature on caesarian sections becomes available more women are choosing to have epidurals in favour of general anaesthetic caesarians. With an epidural the mother is awake, alert and breathing on her own, as opposed to a general anaesthetic caesarian where the mother's breathing is performed by a ventilator. The obvious benefit to medical staff, apart from the safety aspects, is the opportunity to be able to communicate with the couple throughout the procedure.

OBSTETRICIAN

With a caesarian done under epidural anaesthesia we must block half way up the ribcage to the vertebrae just under the bust and down to the bottom of the pelvis to numb the lining of the inside of the abdomen.

ANAESTHETIST

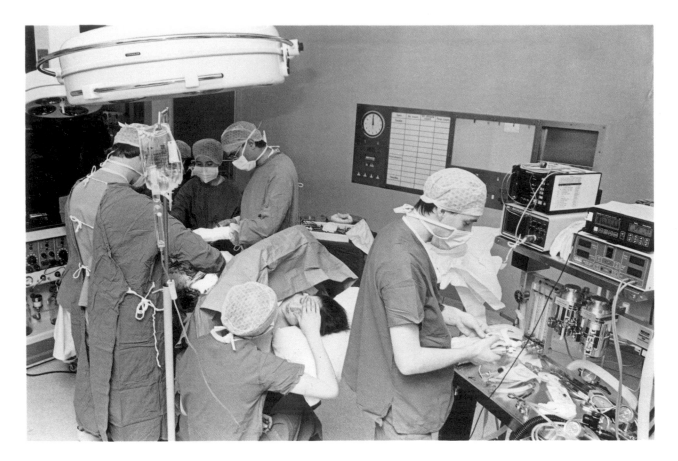

It nearly finished me off when I entered the operating theatre – seeing the lights and the instruments all set up. I felt very dizzy and queasy. The anaesthetist gave me something which relieved the queasy feeling immediately.

The anaesthetist tested various parts of the abdomen to make sure that the area was numb. In spite of this I had in the back of my mind the fear that I might feel something during the operation, and that the anaesthetic might wear off before the operation was finished. Ken was so comforting which alleviated some of my anxieties.

LESLEY

The dizzy, queasy feeling is caused by a drop in blood pressure. A drug is given intravenously which squeezes down the blood vessels in the legs and therefore brings the blood pressure up, relieving the queasy feeling. We monitor her pulse rate, the amount of oxygen she is getting into her blood and her blood pressure throughout the caesarian. In spite of having the operation under epidural anaesthesia, the anaesthetic machine is ready at hand in the event that we had to convert to a general caesarian.

ANAESTHETIST

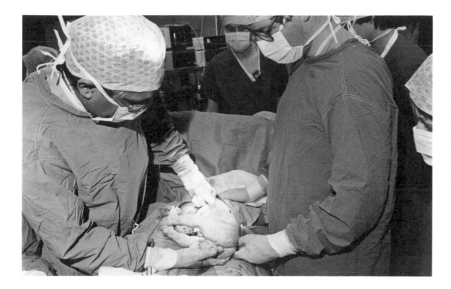

The baby's bottom has just been delivered. I am delivering the left arm by cradling the upper section of the arm. I hold it up and then deliver the other arm. The important feature here is that I am gently applying traction to the baby's bottom, and that at no stage is the baby's abdomen handled, because the baby's abdominal structures are so delicate and likely to be traumatised.

OBSTETRICIAN

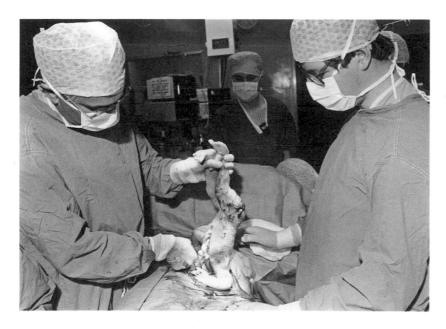

This baby is an extended breech where the baby's legs are stretched out with the feet near the shoulders. With the legs extended into the air, I ease a finger into the baby's mouth and gently extend the head and the baby is delivered.

OBSTETRICIAN

As the baby was being delivered I could feel pulling and pushing in my abdomen but it was less painful than having the baby kicking inside me.

LESLEY

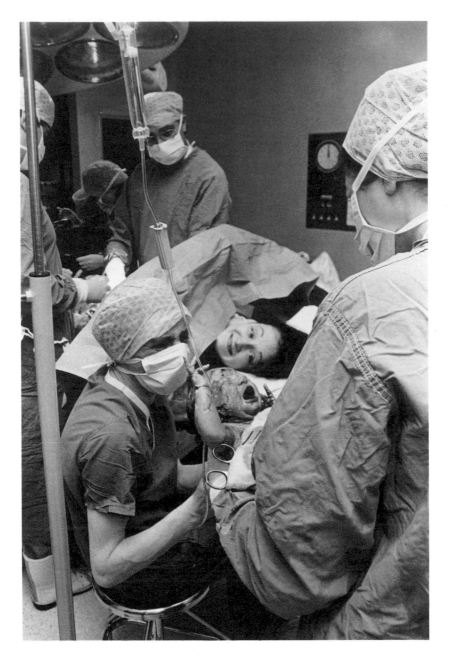

I remember someone saying, 'It's a
boy' and hearing an awful lot of
crying, I didn't realise he was out
until he was appearing by my left
shoulder. I was totally stunned and
Ken burst into tears.

LESLEY

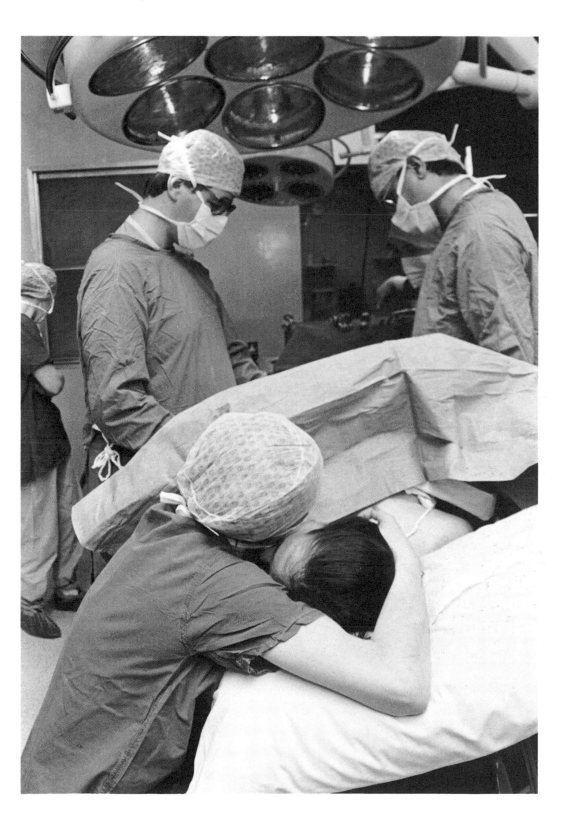

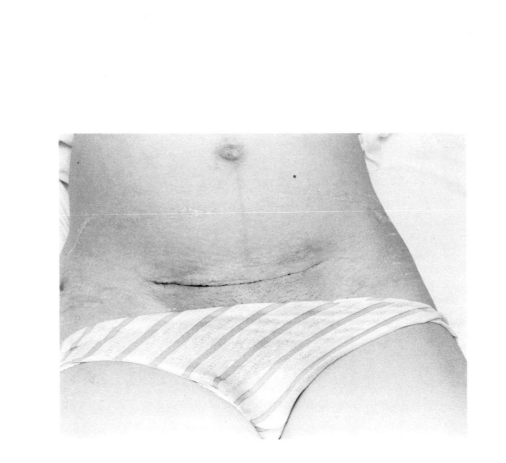

Three day old scar – the stitches are
self-dissolving.

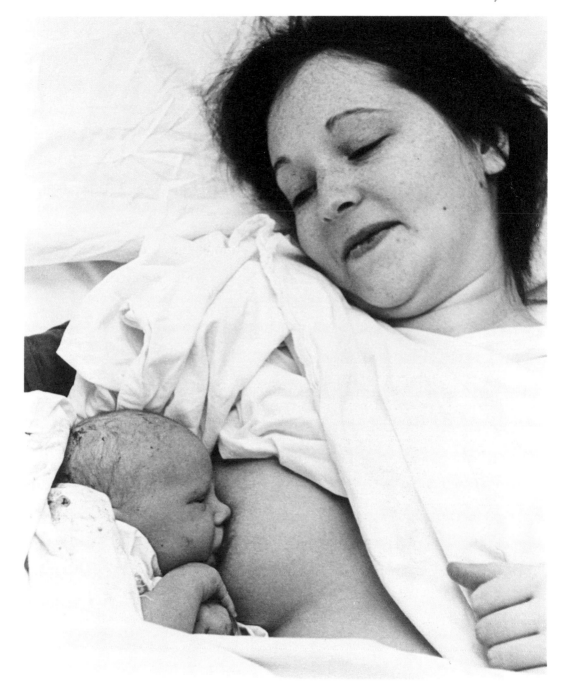

Most parents' main concern is whether the baby has everything . . . two arms, two legs, ten toes . . . You can't answer the parents unless you have had a good look . . . often the pediatrician will check the cord, suck the mucus out from the baby, dry and wrap the baby and then bring the baby to the parents. The mother can hold the baby while she is being stitched up.

If one believes in bonding, the process begins right here – another advantage of having an epidural caesarian.

OBSTETRICIAN

With these
final pushes there was a
strange feeling that even when
you have finished pushing
the pushing continues in
spite of yourself, overriding
what you are doing.

HELEN

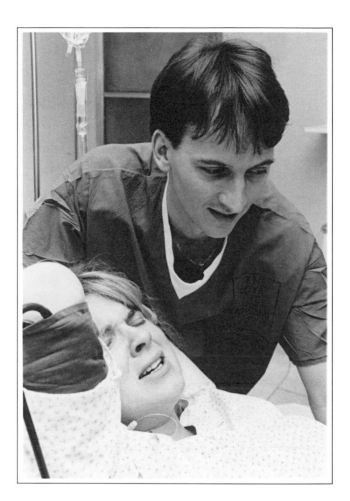

Helen and Paul

Helen is twenty-six years old, first
pregnancy. Her waters broke at 3am at
home while she was sleeping. She had a
vaginal breech delivery at 7.45am in
hospital.

At thirty-five weeks of pregnancy I was diagnosed as having a breech baby – bottom coming first. I went into a panic thinking that's it, I'll need a caesarian. All my plans for an active childbirth had flown out the window. However, I was reassured by the doctor that depending on the size of my pelvis and the size of the baby that I could still have a vaginal delivery.

HELEN

A pelvic x-ray was taken to look at Helen's pelvis and the passage through which the baby would go at the time of delivery, to see if the size of the pelvis was bigger than the baby and therefore would not obstruct the baby's delivery. She had a good sized pelvis and an average sized baby and should therefore have a good vaginal delivery.

From about thirty-five to thirty-six weeks of pregnancy there is a small possibility that the baby will turn around but it's still very likely that it will be a breech delivery. The fluid within the uterus reduces from this stage onwards making less room for the baby to manoeuvre within the uterus.

We recommend having an epidural for a breech delivery – with an epidural one can do a relaxed, controlled delivery of the head. The head is the crucial part of the baby and comes last. This is the one time as the head is descending that the woman has an unbearable urge to push. The danger of this is that the sudden delivery 'pop' of the head produces a situation of compression and sudden decompression which is associated with bleeding within the brain – what we call intraventricular haemorrhage.

Breech labours tend to be longer and more painful (because it's bottom first) so that an epidural makes for a less traumatic experience. It's better to have a woman who is alert, who has had periods of sleep during labour and who is ready to enjoy her baby, rather than a woman who has been given repeated doses of pethidine, becomes zonked out and misses the most magnificent part of the labour which is experiencing the actual birth and ultimately holding the baby. Another advantage of the epidural is that should a decision be made to perform a caesarian section during labour, the operation can be performed under the existing epidural anaesthetic.

OBSTETRICIAN

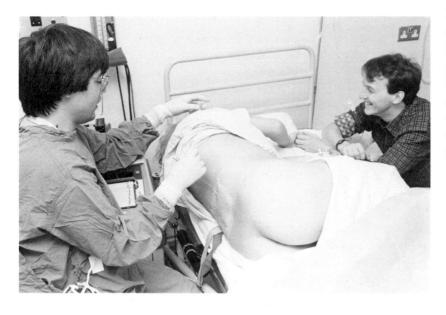

I was feeling tense and aware of everything that was happening to me but the procedure was not really painful. When the needle was first inserted I felt a lot of pressure, then a sensation like an electric shock running down my leg, followed by a tingling, numbing sensation and then shivering.

HELEN

Instituting the epidural block is always done under sterile conditions as one does not want to introduce germs into the spinal column. A needle is inserted between the vertebrae in the lower back into the epidural space which surrounds the spinal cord. A thin plastic tube (catheter) is inserted into the space and the needle removed. A local anaesthetic is injected into the tube which will block the nerve routes supplying the sensations and power to the lower half of the body. The plastic tube is left in place covered in swabs and sticky tape.

Top ups of anaesthetic can be given when necessary through a small bacterial filter conveniently placed in Helen's case over the right shoulder. The time it takes for the anaesthetic to take effect is approximately fifteen to thirty minutes from the time that the plastic tube is in place.

The effects of the epidural will have worn off within one to one and a half hours of the last dose and the mother will be walking within six to eight hours of having given birth.

ANAESTHETIST

Shaking/shivering is a very common consequence of labour, because of hyperventilating before, during and after contractions, and because of the stress of the situation. Hyperventilating (heavy, fast breathing) produces a chemical imbalance in the blood. Shaking/shivering after an epidural is probably due to an increased heat loss as a consequence of the opening of the blood vessels that an epidural produces. The lower half of the body where the epidural is taking effect feels warm while the upper half of the body which has normal temperature control is shaking and shivering in an attempt to conserve heat.

ANAESTHETIST

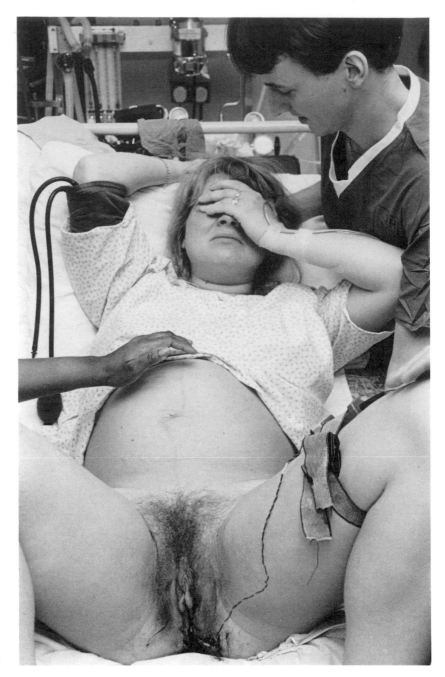

Because it wasn't a very long labour my husband Paul didn't really have to do anything for me. I wouldn't have wanted him to be soothing but I was glad he was at my side and not down at the other end like the medical staff.

HELEN

The foetal scalp electrode is traditionally applied to the scalp but it can also be applied to the baby's bottom. You want one of the electrodes making contact with the foetal skin, so that you can get a good continuous pulse, which reflects the foetal heart rate. Because the breech is a riskier labour than if the head was coming *first, we monitor the foetal heart rate continuously.*

In spite of the fact that Helen's cervix was fully dilated at 5am, Helen did not start pushing until 6.30am. If the cervix is found to be fully dilated and the breech baby is still quite high in the birth canal we don't encourage pushing. We try to ensure that there *are adequate contractions and that the uterus functions well in pushing the baby further down into the pelvis. We allow the breech to descend right on to the perineum to the point where if you part the labia you can just about see the baby's bottom and then we get the mother pushing.*

OBSTETRICIAN

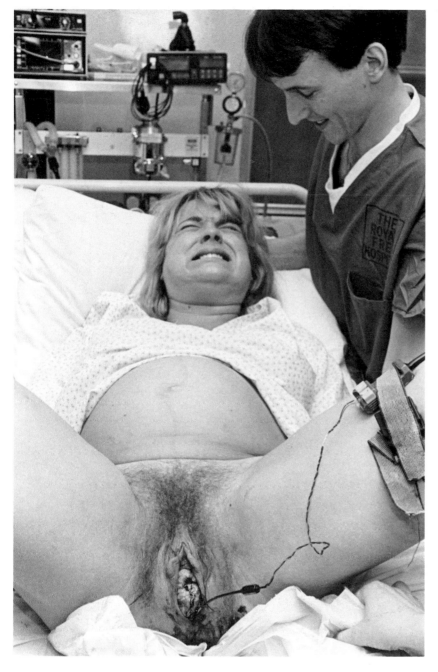

The bottom is just visible. The labia are parted and the perineum stretched.
OBSTETRICIAN

At about 6.30am. I felt a deep pain at the base of the pubic area and I wanted to push.

HELEN

You want to block the painful part of contractions without blocking all sensation, you want the woman to feel a little niggle or tightening with contractions so that she is aware of what is going on and is not totally numb from the waist down. It's not always possible. There is a huge variation between woman to woman in how they react to the epidural.

Helen was able to push without feeling the full discomfort at the perineal end. When she received a top up of anaesthetic she was sitting up so that it was the perineum which became numb, not the abdomen and she could feel to push.

ANAESTHETIST

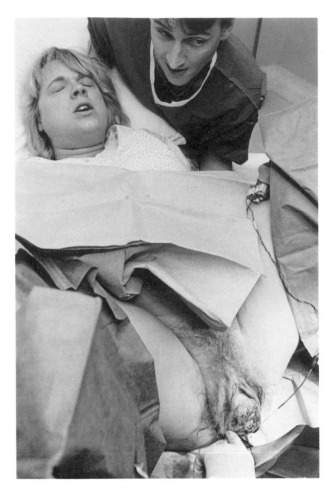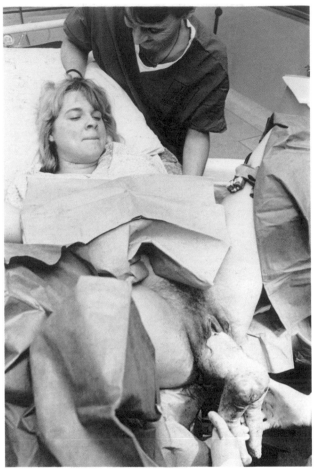

The baby's bottom has appeared beyond the vagina. An index finger is inserted on Helen's right side parting the labia. It is not always necessary to do this as the baby's buttocks can push the labia open themselves. Just prior to this stage an episiotomy was performed. It widens the outlet so that there is less of a compressed effect on the baby.

OBSTETRICIAN

The baby has come out unaided. This is an example of an extended breech where the legs have been right up alongside of the body and the feet are on either side of the baby's ears. The baby comes out like this. To deliver the legs we place a thumb behind each knee so that the knee bends enabling the delivery of both legs. The mother then pushes with the next contraction and the baby descends further.

OBSTETRICIAN

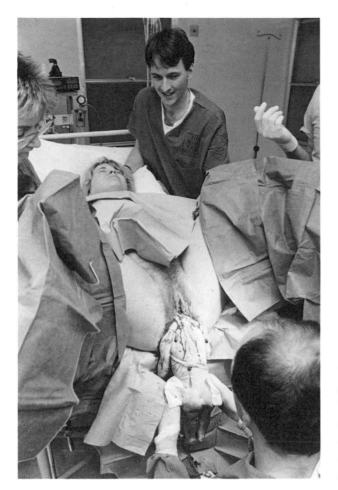

With these final pushes there was a strange feeling that even when you have finished pushing the pushing continues in spite of yourself, overriding what you are doing. I felt a tugging each time a leg or arm came out.

HELEN

Both arms have now been delivered. The cord is around the baby and the baby is being supported. It is important to make sure that the cord continues pulsating throughout the delivery thus assuring that the baby is getting a constant blood supply from the placenta. The cord is still intact, the baby is not yet breathing and is entirely dependent on its mother for oxygen. If the cord stops pulsating there is then a need to deliver the baby quickly although this is a very rare occurrence.

I can just see the nape of the baby's neck, Helen is still pushing. This is an ideal situation – a cooperative, relaxed mother and no evident foetal distress.

OBSTETRICIAN

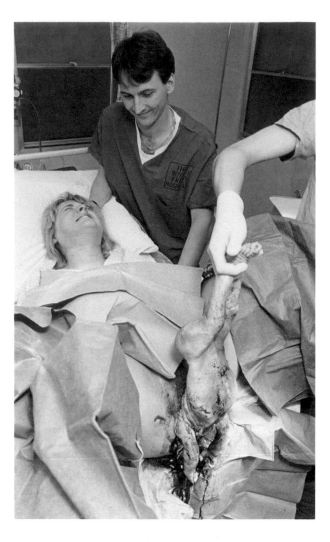

The assistant has grasped both ankles and has raised the baby upwards, being careful not to hyperextend – not to bend the spine and neck too much.

OBSTETRICIAN

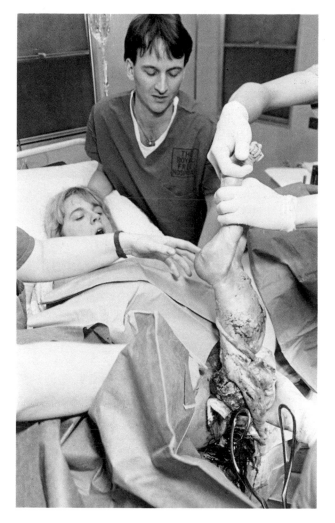

Forceps were applied to the baby's head and the head gently delivered. The forceps function as a guide and a protective cage around the baby's head.
OBSTETRICIAN

This is a sutured 2″ medio-lateral episiotomy.

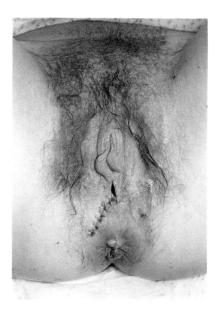

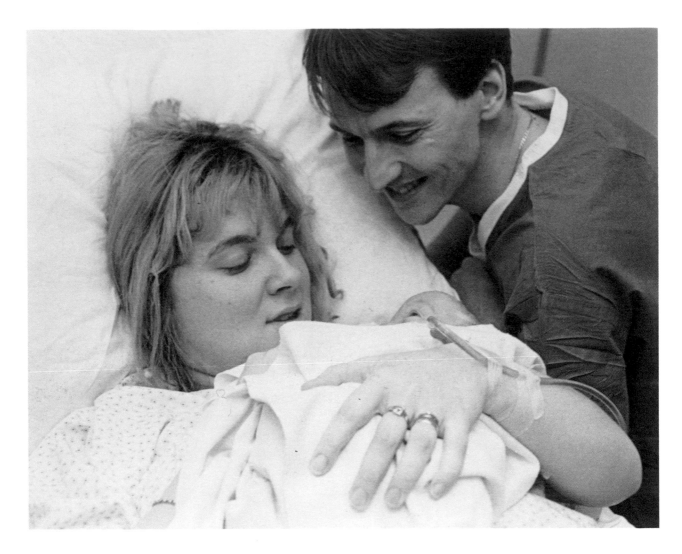

My first feeling when I held her –
elated but shattered.

HELEN

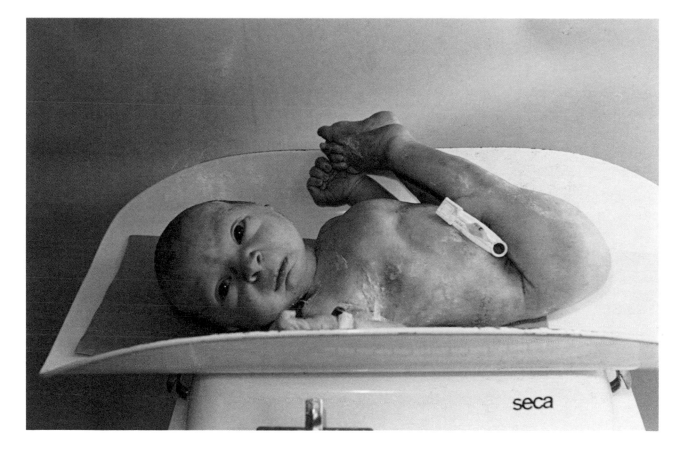

This represents exactly the position of
the baby in utero. The legs usually
straighten within a day or two,
sometimes almost immediately.

OBSTETRICIAN

Such a feeling
of amazement. It's a strange
feeling to be amazed, but up
to a point one is giving birth
to a head, and then it's
a little baby lying there . . .
Look what I have done.

LEISHA

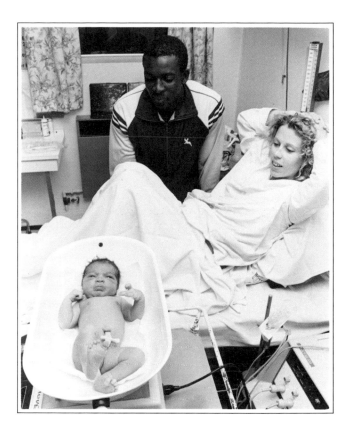

Leisha
and Aiden

Leisha is twenty-five years old, first
pregnancy. She went into labour early
evening on her due date. After an active
labour Zawadi was born at 5.45am.

After eight years of being on the pill, I fell pregnant just three days after I had stopped taking the pill. Even before I started getting any symptoms like sore breasts, I knew that I was pregnant. I went into the newsagent's and found myself looking at a pregnancy book. I was so shocked at what I had done that I put the book down and left the shop.

LEISHA

11pm We had friends round and I was making pizzas. Contractions were coming about every fifteen minutes. I found myself crouching through them.

Midnight I had a bath and wanted to try and get a night's sleep but Aiden asked me how I was going to sleep with contractions happening about every five minutes – they were becoming too painful to lie down.

1am I called the hospital. They suggested that perhaps I come in within the hour. It took us that long just to pack our bags. I think Aiden was planning to be there for days. He packed so much food – and never got a chance to eat any of it.

LEISHA

Aiden called me at 1.30am to say that they were leaving for the hospital.

NANCY

3.10am I was examined and told that my cervix was 2cm dilated.
3am–5am We walked the corridors, squatting whenever a contraction came. Aiden supported me from behind and rubbed my belly. He was so calm about everything, breathing with and for me.

LEISHA

I was there to make sure that all went according to the way Leisha had planned – there were times in early labour when she wanted to stop and sit down, but I reminded her that it wasn't what she had intended to do . . . and so we kept moving . . . and squatting when a contraction came. Massaging Leisha's belly felt good for both of us – and I continued to do this up until the pushing.

AIDEN

5am The contractions started getting much closer together. I vomited. The midwife said, 'I think you're going to have this baby, immediately. Hop on this table [which I found difficult] and I'll examine you. Oh! You're 9cm dilated, that was quick' and she whistled me down to the delivery room in a wheelchair.

LEISHA

5.30am As I was fully dilated the midwife broke the membranes to speed things up. A scalp electrode was clipped on the baby's head.

LEISHA

At 5.10am Aiden telephoned to tell me that Leisha was already 9cm dilated. I broke all speed limits to cross London and arrived just as Leisha was feeling the baby's head.

NANCY

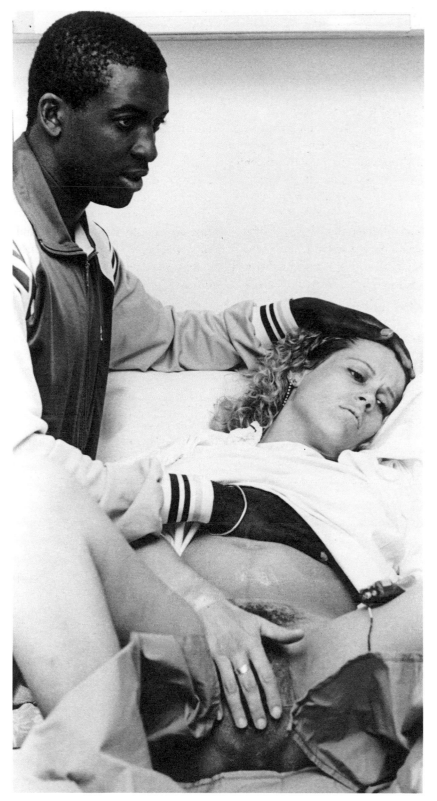

Everyone had built up the transition
stage as being a time when you have
an overwhelming desire to push but
are told not to. I never experienced
this urge to push until the time to
push arrived.

I could feel lots of hair, it
wasn't what I thought it would feel
like – so moist and soft . . . I knew
that the end was near.

LEISHA

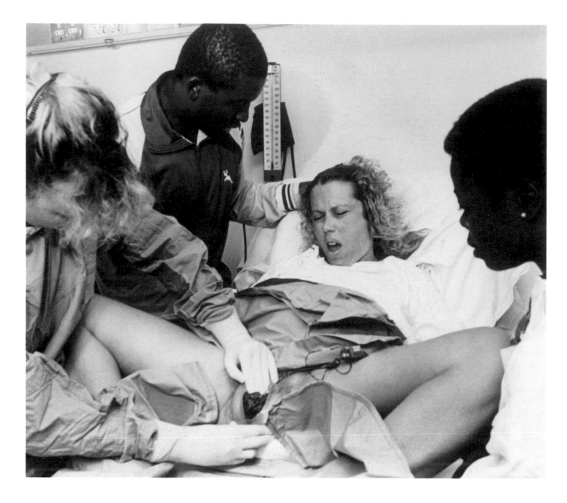

Great relief at the moment when the
head came out, but I don't
remember it as being unpleasant.

LEISHA

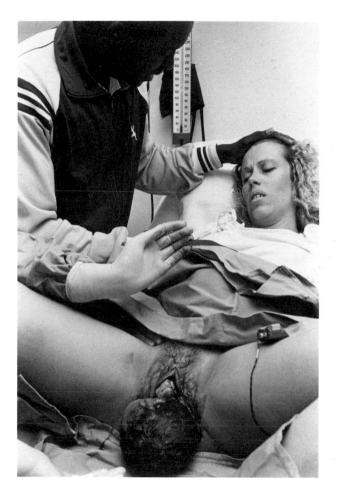

The baby is coming out waving.
The fist is tucked up beside her face.
This is called a compound presentation.
You can try and push the hand down
but in this case it was not successful.
Leisha had small vaginal wall tears.

MIDWIFE

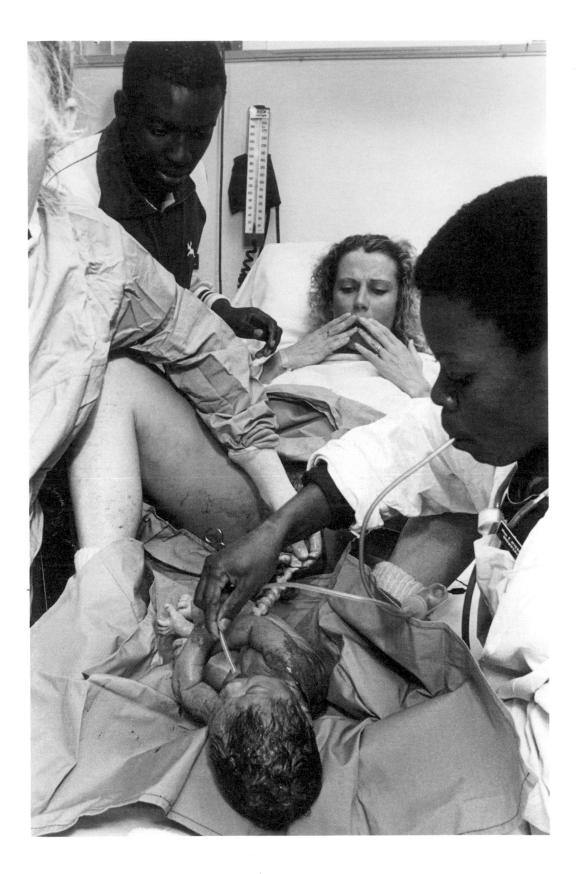

Such a feeling of amazement. It's a strange feeling to be amazed, but up to a point one is giving birth to a head, and then it's a little baby lying there . . . Look what I have done.

LEISHA

At 5.45am Zawadi was born. Zawadi is Swahili for gift.

Breathless, every wonderful word that you could think of – but breathless describes my feeling at that moment. I was very tearful, looking at her.

AIDEN

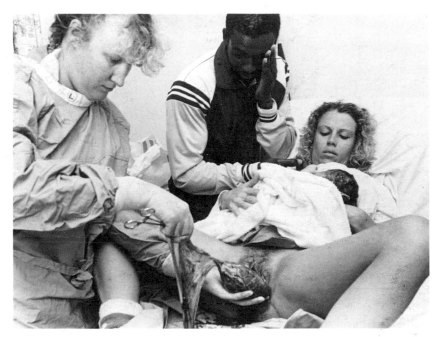

I am delivering the placenta by controlled cord traction. It is important to check that the placenta has come away completely and that none of it has been retained in the uterus. This can be the cause of post partum bleeding. We examine the placenta to ensure that it has two membranes – the amnion and the chorion – and we look at the umbilical cord to make sure that it contains two arteries and a vein.

MIDWIFE

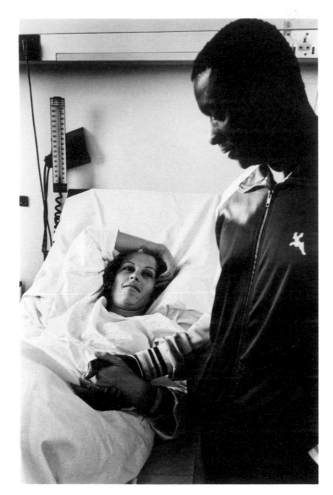

I thought Aiden had the harder job really, I had a definite role. I was there to give birth. Aiden's role was less defined but he did everything – we were doing it together.

LEISHA

A father *has* to be present at the birth. It's a joint event, not something that the woman should have to do on her own. The man was present at the start and should see her through till the end. I was breathing with her from the time contractions began at home, timing and writing them down, packing her bag – the fact that I ended up with backache and a headache was nothing. I did what I had to do.

AIDEN

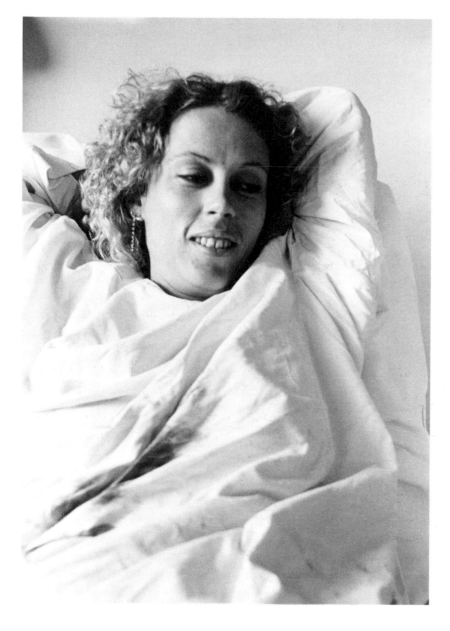

I felt very serene. I felt as if my heart had stopped beating . . . everything was so quiet. It's contentment. I have never felt so at one with myself.

LEISHA

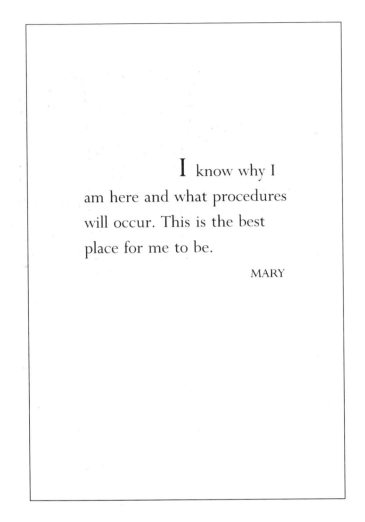

I know why I am here and what procedures will occur. This is the best place for me to be.

MARY

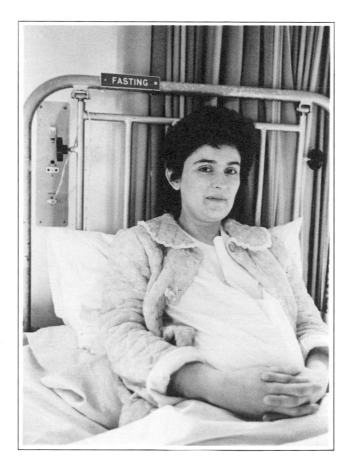

Mary

Mary is thirty-seven years old. She has five children and has had three miscarriages. This baby has rhesus disease of the newborn and was delivered by caesarian section at thirty-two weeks.

During Mary's earlier pregnancies she developed antibodies to a component of the baby's red blood cells which were inherited from the father. Mary's blood is rhesus negative but her husband and her baby are rhesus positive. Rhesus disease of the newborn can be prevented provided that the rhesus negative woman whose partner is rhesus positive is given an injection after the first delivery. This ensures that she will not become sensitised and develop antibodies in later pregnancies. Mary was not given this injection after her first delivery.

With this pregnancy amniocentesis was performed at sixteen weeks. There was evidence of severe red blood cell destruction as the foetus was affected by rhesus disease. With this information it was decided to perform a caesarian section at thirty-two weeks.

OBSTETRICIAN

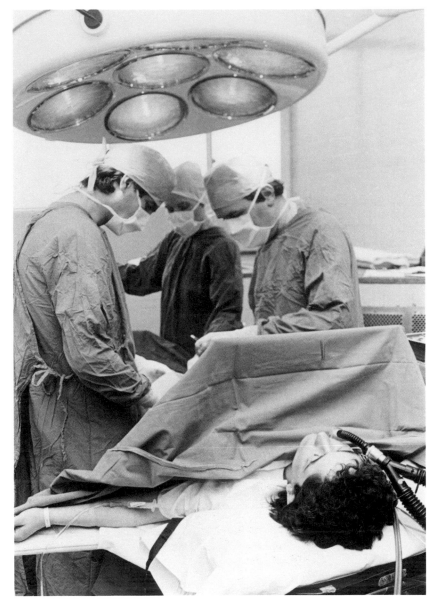

I know why I am here and what procedures will occur. This is the best place for me to be. Joseph, my five-year-old was delivered by caesarian section at thirty weeks. He needed five blood exchanges . . . but he's grand now, not a bother on him.

My husband is very worried. He's home looking after the children. All that matters to us is that this baby is alive.

MARY

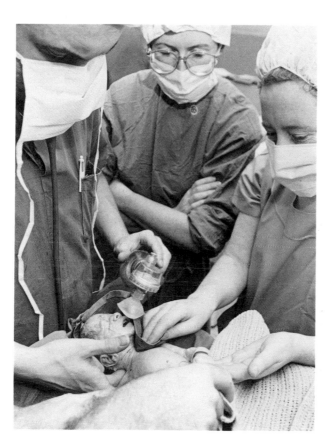

A baby this young should be very pink. This baby is pale, a sign that the red blood cell count is low. It is because he is a rhesus baby and the mother's rhesus antibodies are destroying the baby's red blood cells. It is therefore necessary to remove his blood which contains antibodies and give him fresh blood with no antibodies. This is done with an exchange transfusion which replaces approximately two-thirds of the baby's blood.

PEDIATRICIAN

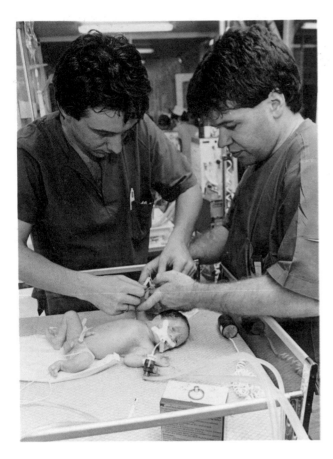

This baby was eight weeks pre term and will most likely be in the special care baby unit for seven to eight weeks. He will probably be quite sick for the first few days but should improve quickly. With a premature baby respiration is often a problem as the lungs are not yet fully developed. Because this was a planned operation the baby was given some steroids, which some people argue will decrease the incidence of lung disease, so we might hope to get him off the ventilator by the end of the first week.

The babies usually lose some weight as it takes a while to establish them on full feeds. By two to three weeks we hope that he would have regained his birth weight of 3lb 10oz and by three to four weeks he should weigh between 5lb 2oz and 5lb 7oz. That is how it should go but we have a lot of mountains to cross and there are many possible complications.

PEDIATRICIAN

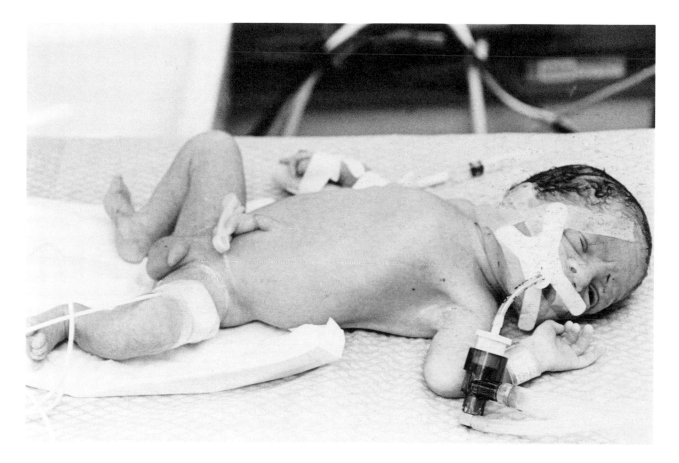

Baby Don Martin returned home at
five weeks weighing 5lb 2oz. He had
received two blood exchanges. He is
now thriving.

I am really,
really, really pleased you are
here Gareth. It makes all the
difference in the world you
holding me . . . you have no
idea.

JEAN

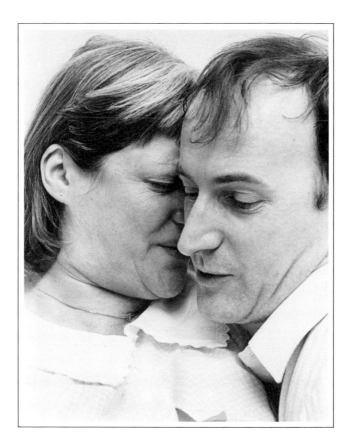

Jean and Gareth

Jean is forty years old, first pregnancy.
She and Gareth had been trying to have
a baby for three years and succeeded as
part of a study trial. Jean's labour was
induced at forty weeks.

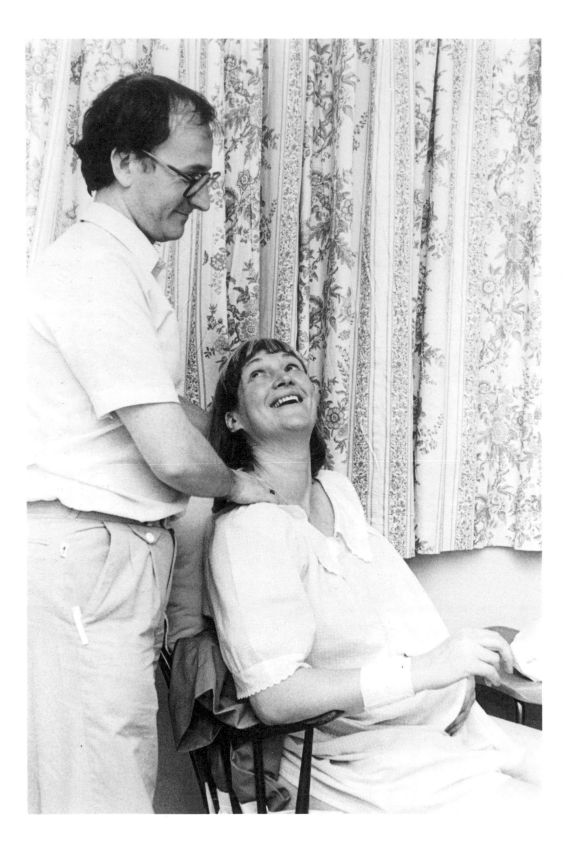

We had been trying for a baby for three years. I never prayed for a baby while I was trying to conceive because we thought if I wasn't conceiving there was a reason. We also thought that if we didn't ask God for a baby there was a chance of a 'maybe'. But if we asked, He might just say no. However, close friends in our church study group finally convinced us to begin praying and we regularly prayed, 'Please, please, please God let me have a baby, and if I cannot, let me bear not having one'. I did relax and become more philosophical about it.

And then we had the good fortune to be part of a study trial called LIPSI – Laparoscopic Intra Peritoneal Seminal Injection – for couples who have no apparent reasons for not conceiving. The only unnatural bit was being given an artificial period on a given date so that fourteen days later I ovulated on the day when the operating theatre was available for this procedure – in our case on a Wednesday. Under general anaesthetic, a small incision was made in my umbilicus, Gareth's 'washed' sperm were then injected into my peritoneal cavity under direct vision with a laparoscope. The sperm were sprayed around the two ripe eggs, which had not yet burst, and around the top of the uterus as well as being injected vaginally. The surgeon then burst the follicle containing the eggs – rather like the thin skin that forms on the yolk of a cooked egg – and we waited. Fourteen days later I had a spot of blood and I thought, oh no! But several hours later no more blood and the next day there was still no blood. I waited several days but was so impatient that I bought a pregnancy indicator kit. It was negative. I wasn't mortified, but I did feel exactly as I feel before my period starts. I rang up the doctor of the LIPSI trial who told me not to believe my results and to come in for a scan, and there it was, this minute blob   the doctors were hopping up and down excitedly and I cried, tears of joy. We were the first couple to have succeeded on this trial.

JEAN

123

When I was full term my labour was induced using a prostaglandin pessary. I would have liked to have waited another twenty-four hours to see whether the 3.00am twinges and mucus shows would have progressed into labour. But being forty years old, and my first pregnancy a special one, they didn't want to take any chances.

We spent the morning and afternoon walking in the corridors and keeping mobile. The contractions were very bearable.

At 5.00pm an internal examination indicated that my cervix was 2cm dilated. They broke my waters and inserted a scalp electrode. This was excruciatingly painful . . . in fact vaginal examinations in labour were more painful than the contractions.

I was very disappointed when Ruth, my midwife, said they were going to put up a drip, I had such negative feelings about the drip and thought that if they were using a drip things must be going wrong, but I thought brace up Jean this is not a time to get upset now.

JEAN

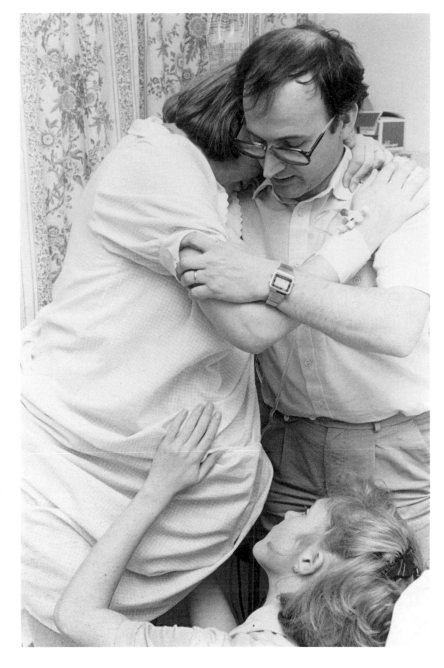

We decided to put Jean on a syntocinon drip. Syntocinon is a hormone which brings about contractions in a woman who is not contracting or augments the contractions that are there. In Jean's case she began contracting every two to three minutes.

MIDWIFE

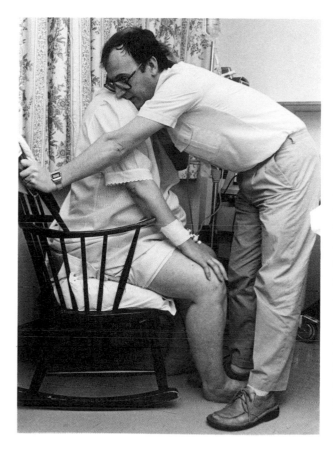

I had an injection of pethidine because I didn't know how bad the contractions were going to be and I didn't want to be agitated by the pain. I wanted everything to be as normal as was possible and therefore taking the pethidine I thought would enable me to do that . . . and I did not want an epidural. I wanted to feel the baby being born and to be in control when I needed to push – true, the pain would be obliterated with an epidural but so would my experience. Pethidine didn't take away the pain. It did make me marginally high but I was euphoric anyway.

My legs felt wonky, but I wanted to stand. When I stood up it helped to ease the contractions but my legs wouldn't hold me. Sitting on a bed pan in a rocking chair kept the pressure off the perineum.

JEAN

I am really, really, really pleased you
are here Gareth. It makes all the
difference in the world you holding
me . . . you have no idea.

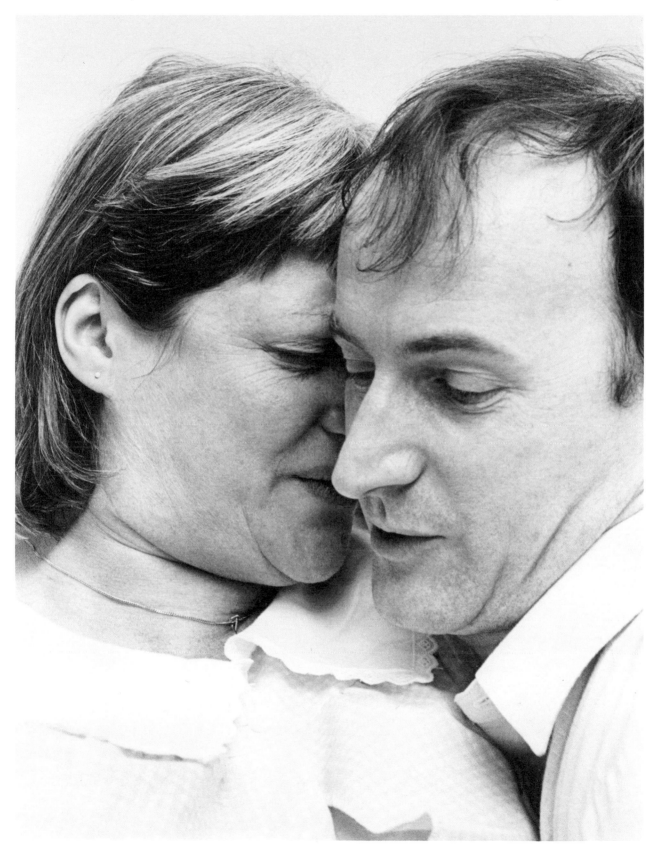

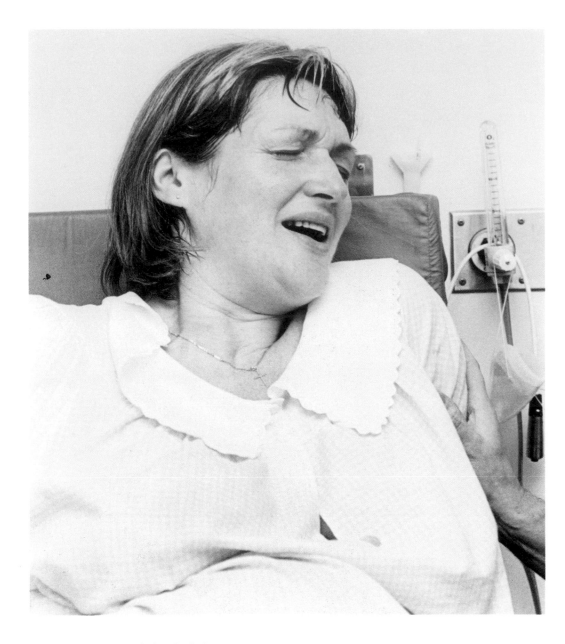

O. . . ooooo. . . that feels a little bit
sexy. I don't mean in a lascivious
way, I mean literally the beautiful
aspect of sex was in my mind
throughout, it's all to do with having
this baby, loving Gareth and being
there together. After one contraction
there was a feeling of an orgasm
with it – something taking hold of
my abdomen and pushing it, an
orgasm without the niceness. I was a
bit surprised by the feeling.

JEAN

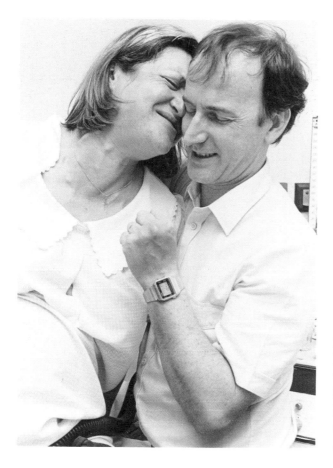

I can't say how much Gareth helped. It sounds corny to go on about it but to have that person who you know best in the world to hang on to, to listen to, to remind you of practical things, like putting your chin down on your chest to push . . .

JEAN

A. . . a. . . a. . . a. . . agh.
I thought who made that sound? It
was a strange spontaneous sound.
Just before that sound I didn't
believe that the baby was so near, I
thought that you were all chivvying
me along – even when Ruth brought
my hand down, it didn't feel like his
head and I thought, 'Oh no I have
felt the wrong bit – never mind',
then a horrid stinging feeling took
over, but it made me push harder to
get rid of it. I knew that it was
because the head was at its widest
point. I did think that I might split
in two, that I wasn't going to be able
to accommodate this baby . . .

                              JEAN

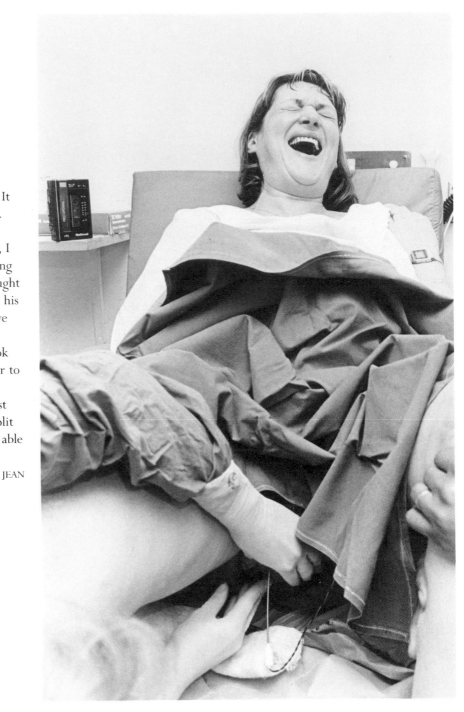

I heard Ruth saying, 'Hello baby'. I noticed Ruth then. She looked serious, 'Jean, we've got to get this baby out now.' I heard a murmur of forceps . . . and thought 'not on your life'. I didn't want me to be cut and him yanked out in such an undignified manner unless it was absolutely necessary. I knew that I had enough energy left to push him out.

JEAN

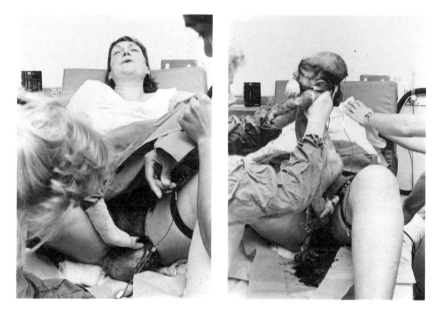

I felt guilty by association because I was unable to take any of the pain from Jean. It was going to be my baby as well and yet I wasn't able to do anything physically to share the pain – yes I could pour iced water and I was glad to help in whatever way I could but I felt inept. I would gladly have shared the pain of contractions. When the baby was born a good dose of the relief that I felt and the tears that I shed were that Jean was no longer in pain. We must have grown closer together by a quantum leap – something we didn't think was possible. We had shared an earth-shattering experience.

GARETH

I'd always kept at bay the idea of holding a baby in my arms . . . until today . . . a protection in case we lost the baby – I couldn't believe that there he was. He is with us and he is ours . . . I am complete now.

JEAN

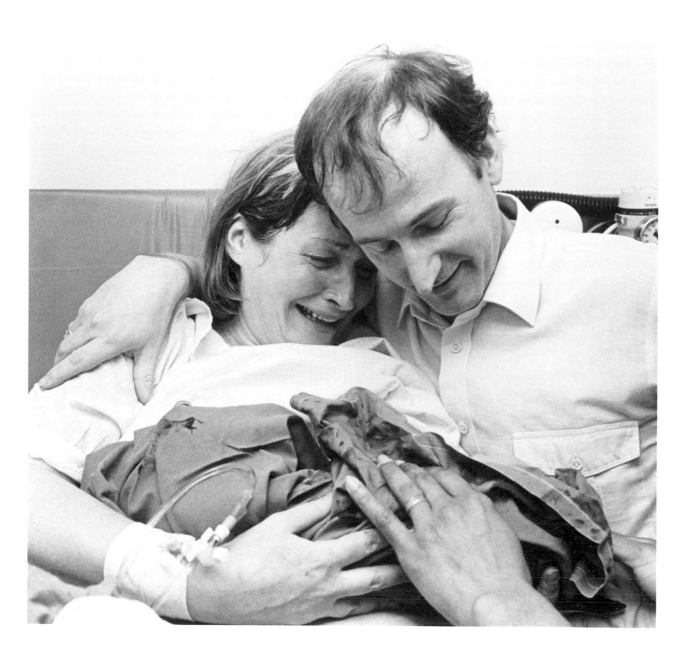

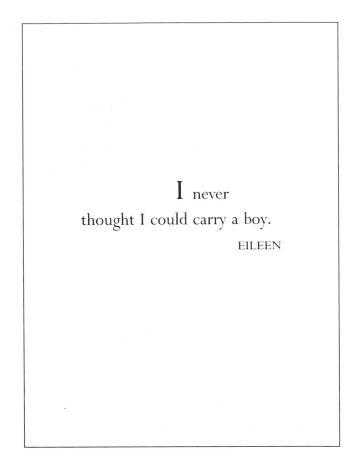

I never
thought I could carry a boy.

EILEEN

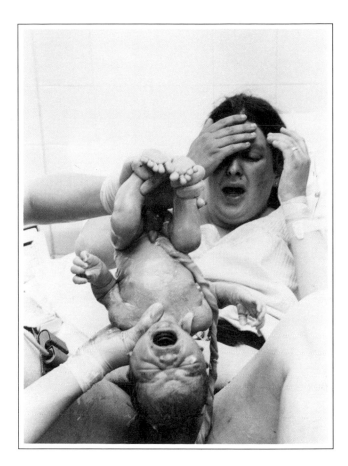

Eileen

Eileen is twenty-six years old, fifth pregnancy. She has had two miscarriages. Her husband was home looking after their two daughters aged five and three.

When I was having contractions at home this morning, my daughter asked, 'Is it hurting the belly off you, mummy?' I would now answer 'Yes', and I have such pains in my legs as if someone were hitting them with a hammer.

I am feeling a little bit nervous. It's been three years since my last birth and last year I lost a baby when I was six months pregnant. It was difficult for my five-year-old daughter. She had told everyone that mummy was going to have a baby and when I went to the hospital and lost the baby, it was very upsetting for her. My mother told her that the baby had died and had gone to heaven. 'Is the baby happy in heaven?' she asked. 'Yes, the baby is with other little girls and boys who have died and she is being looked after by her two great nannies.'

EILEEN

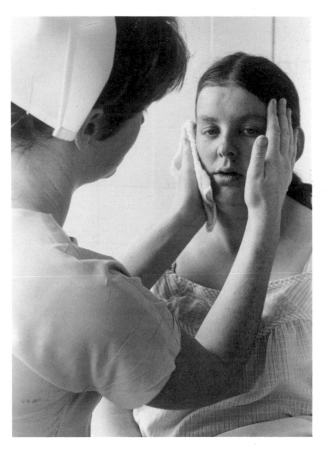

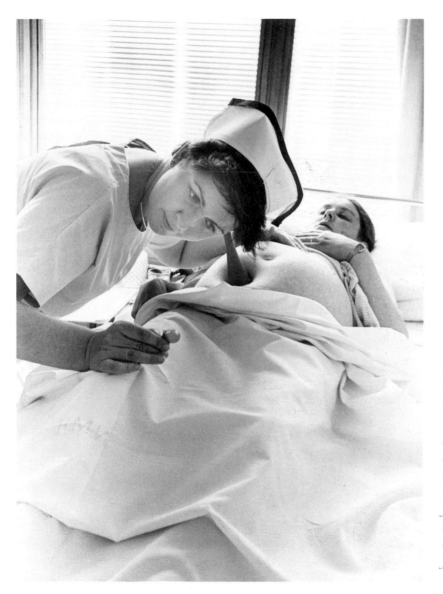

'Auscultating' or listening to the foetal heart is a very important part of the care. This is the only time we deliberately turn away from the woman. Our facial expressions can strongly influence the mother and subconscious (or conscious) frowns on our faces in this situation could unnecessarily worry her. During the first stage of labour the foetal heart is listened to every fifteen minutes, and during the second stage of labour following every contraction.

SISTER

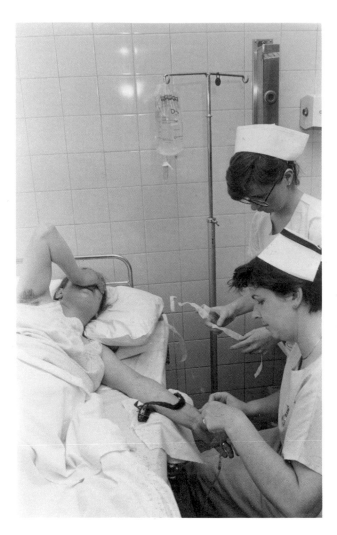 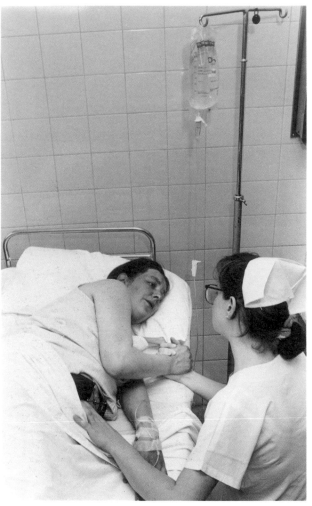

After five hours in labour the uterus was not contracting efficiently. Eileen was only 2-3cm dilated, but getting tired and frustrated. We would expect with a third baby that she would have progressed more quickly than that. The baby's position was perfect. A syntocinon intravenous drip was erected to make contractions more efficient. The number of drops was monitored closely. The drip was left infusing until the delivery was completed.

SISTER

I am terrified of needles because of a very bad childhood experience.

EILEEN

I am reassuring Eileen. When the baby's head is coming down there is so much pressure on the rectum and anus that there is a feeling of having to empty one's bowels – which often happens – it's one of a woman's greater fears.

MIDWIFE

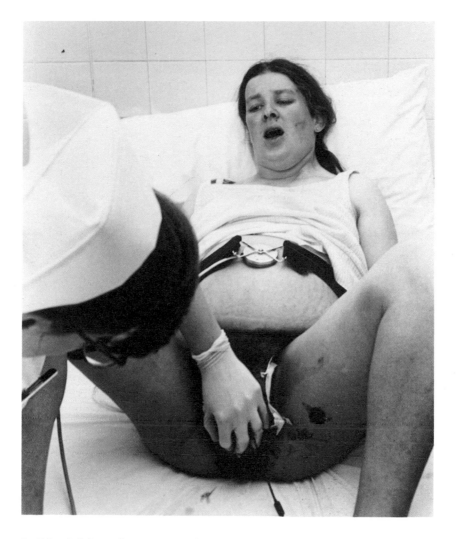

In Eileen's labour the syntocinon drip
brought about the delivery within an
hour. It happened so quickly that there
was no time to remove the foetal heart
monitor straps.

MIDWIFE

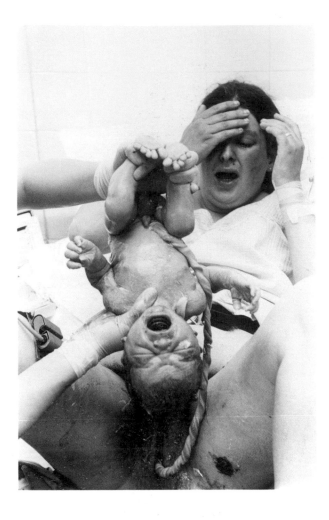

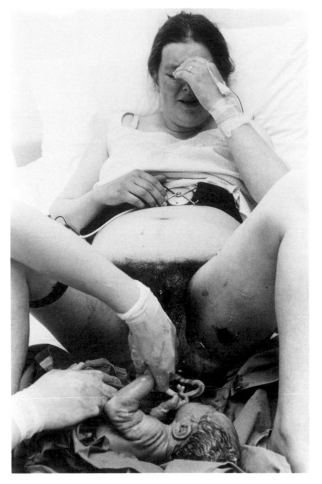

I never thought I could carry a boy.

EILEEN

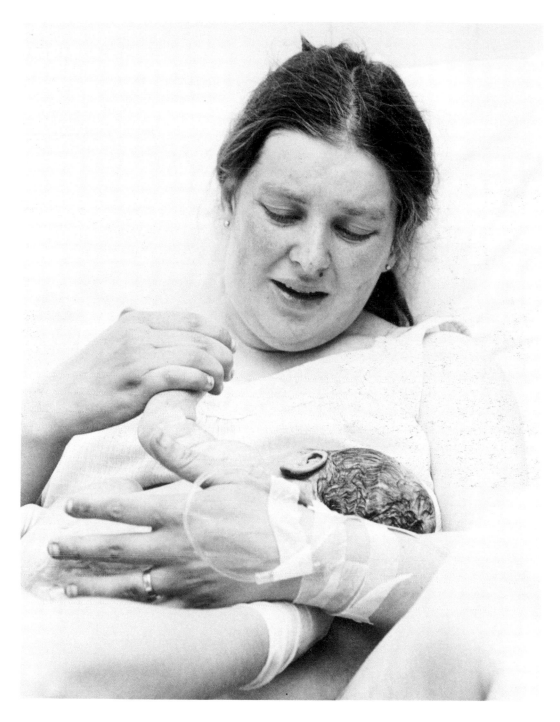

*Eileen's expression says it all, the look
on her face, the gentle touch. This is
just the beginning.*

SISTER

Giving birth in water
was easier than dry birthing . . . Being in our
own home in the presence of trusted friends
felt good. This is easily overlooked and yet
is so very important.

SUE

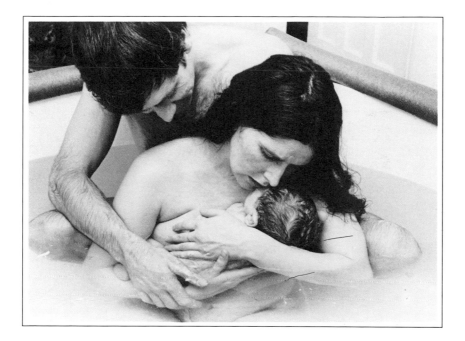

Sue and Ian

Sue is thirty-one years old, second
pregnancy. She had planned for a
home birth the first time but after a
long ordeal was transferred to
hospital. This time she felt better
prepared in herself and knew that
her baby wanted to be born in water.

My joyful child, my little red dragon. During the birth of our daughter Jasemin, I was afraid. I didn't know about riding energy and I didn't know what to expect and I wanted to know. This time I made a choice to be strong, to flow with the powerful birthing energy. Whatever the sensations were they were not going to last forever, I just had to go with them. I made positive affirmations which helped me enormously; programming my mind with my intentions, such as 'It is safe for me to have my perfect healthy baby, at the perfect time, in the perfect way, with the perfect people'.

I knew that our baby wanted to be born in a tank of water at home. This I intuited.

The water has its own energy which is vital, alive and flowing. I'm happy in water, it's where I grew.

Labour began very gently mid afternoon. I repeated out loud to myself the affirmation I had made.

SUE

144

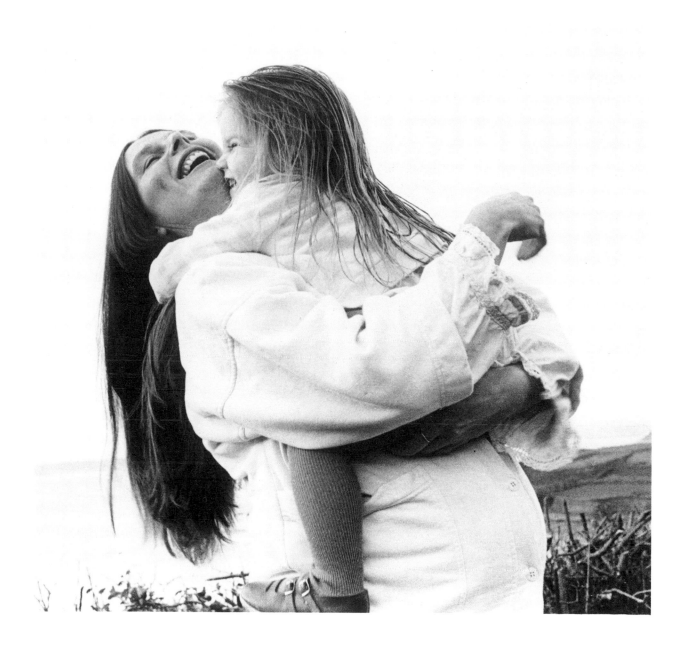

Linked with Ian and Jill my
compassionate surrogate mum.
I was breathing deeply and focusing
my attention into the pelvic area.
The logical, analytical side of my
brain switched off. Time had no
meaning. I didn't communicate apart
from simple directions. I had no
thoughts. I was responding to the
sensations of my body.

SUE

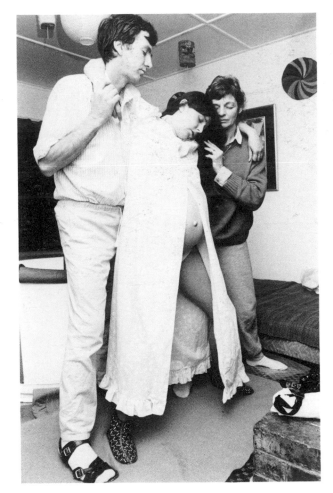

Sue was dealing so well with the
contractions – no complaining, no
wasting of energy, just focusing all
her energies downwards. Sue had
prepared herself physically and
mentally for this birth – she had
come to terms with her fears
surrounding Jasemin's birth. Instead
of resisting the contractions and so
creating tension and pain, she was
relaxing and letting her body get on
with the task of giving birth.

IAN

Late evening our doctor, Roger,
examined me. My cervix was 1cm
dilated. During the early hours of
the morning I practised squatting
and rotating my pelvis rocking from
side to side, generally staying
upright. Lying down was too painful.
At 6am Roger examined me again.
My cervix was only 2cm dilated so
he returned home feeling that we
still had quite a time to go. I said the
baby would be born at 9am. About
6.30am I was sick, my waters broke
and the contractions heated up.

SUE

146

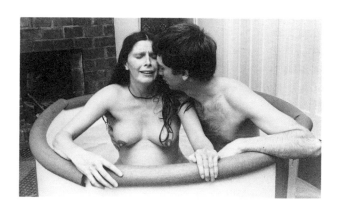

At 8.30am we got into the tank. The water felt warm and luxurious. There was a moment of conflict when I was trying not to push but my body said 'Go!'.

SUE

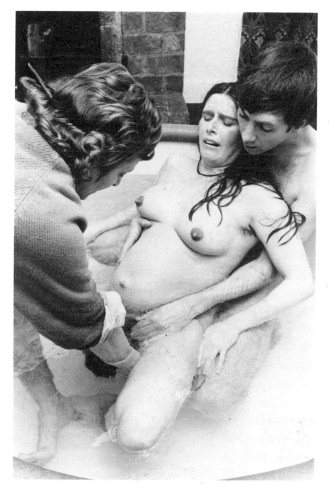

I had a pattern of pushing; making deep grunting sounds followed by gentler breathing and rest between pushes. Then I pushed and roared like a tiger and out came the baby's head. It felt so good to *push* him out.

SUE

I had the reservation that there might be a cord around the neck (my two babies had been born with their cords around their necks). I didn't want to project my anxiety on to Sue. I was not frightened but the danger lights were up a little – the crown of the head was filling the vagina so completely that I couldn't see how I could possibly feel for the cord.

JILL

Roger had not yet arrived. I took over at this point, felt the lie of the head and attempted to feel for any cord around the neck. What an extraordinary feeling . . . those little folds of neck fat but certainly nothing constricting, or so I prayed. With my hands around the baby's chin I waited for Sue's next push.

NANCY

About 2-3 minutes passed which seemed like an eternity. The baby slipped out so easily. I brought him through the water and on to Sue's chest. He cried instantly – what a relief for me to hear that clear cry. I picked up my camera and started photographing only to realise that my camera was covered in vernix from my hands.

NANCY

Aaron was born at 9am. I took Aaron's little body in my arms and comforted him. He was crying. I think he wanted to stay underwater longer. During the next half hour we lay back and relaxed in the warm water with our little man Aaron.

SUE

The water in the tank is body temperature – 37.2°C (98.6°F) – with this fibre glass insulated tub measuring 4ft wide by 2ft 6in deep you lose approximately 1°C of heat every hour. You can top up the temperature by pouring a kettle of hot water into the tank. The room temperature should be very warm.

Providing that the baby has not yet surfaced and providing that the placenta is still functioning and the blood is still being pumped through the cord to the baby the baby can stay underwater indefinitely. I have never known a baby not to be all right for twenty to thirty minutes. The baby usually sinks because its lungs are not filled with air.

In general I bring the baby quite quickly out of the water. The argument for leaving the baby floating in the water is that it is akin to being in utero – which it is – but a baby floating inside the mother is surrounded by mother. It feels the pressure of the womb and is in contact with the mother's own energy fields. I think that it might get a bit lonely floating in the water on its own so I tend to bring the baby on to the mother's tummy if she is lying on her back or into her arms if she is squatting. I have not yet delivered a water baby who has had any difficulty taking its first breath. I feel that it is because I don't use pethidine or gas and air. Water removes much of the pain of childbirth.

ROGER

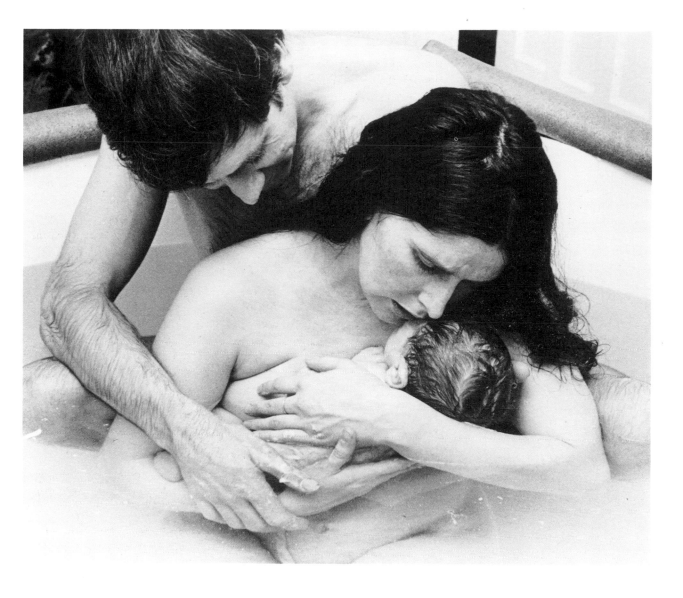

Shortly after Roger arrived (9.20am) I had the urge to push the placenta out. Roger clamped and cut the cord and with one push the placenta was expelled. We buried the placenta in the garden under a tree so that it may continue to give life.

SUE

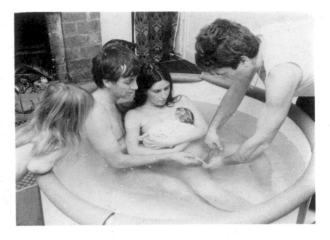

I gave Sue a dose of arnica to take. Arnica is a homeopathic remedy used where bruising of soft tissue has occurred. The birth canal has been bruised and stretched as the baby descended. Arnica will help to heal the internal bruising.

ROGER

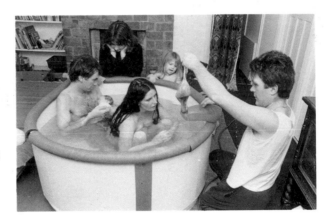

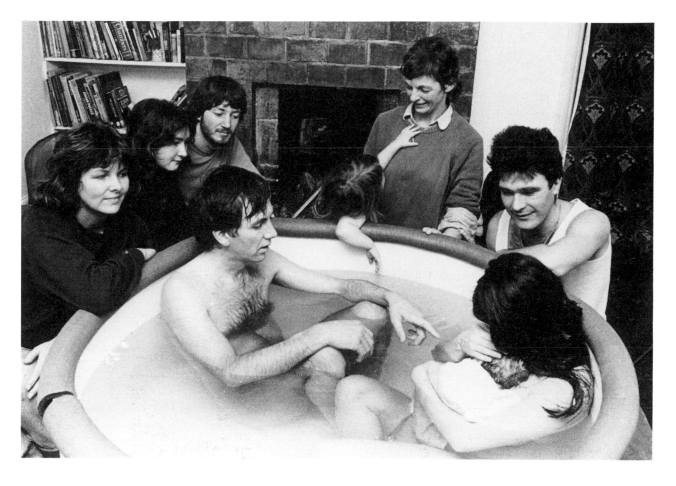

Giving birth in water was easier than dry birthing. The relaxing environment of the warm water removed much of the downward pressure of the baby as he moved through the birth canal. I did not tear.

SUE

Being in our own home in the presence of trusted friends felt good. This is so easily overlooked and yet is so very important.

SUE AND IAN

'Emma, how can you joke about such a serious matter.' Sunday wouldn't believe that I was pregnant.

EMMA

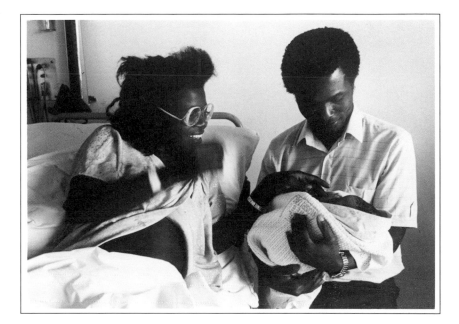

Emma and Sunday

Emma is thirty-two years old, first
pregnancy. She and Sunday had been
trying to conceive for five years. Two
weeks early her waters broke at home at
5.55am and their son was born six hours
later.

Sunday and I had been trying to conceive for five years. A laparoscopy showed that my fallopian tubes were beyond repair. They were full of adhesions, possibly due to an infection in my adolescence of which I was unaware. We became part of the in vitro fertilisation programme but the first three attempts were unsuccessful. Sunday never gave up hope of having a baby even when I had despaired.

First attempt The surgeon was able to collect my eggs but they did not fertilise and therefore were not put back.

Second attempt They were able to collect the eggs, but the eggs were post mature. They did not attempt to fertilise them.

Third attempt They collected the eggs, fertilised them, and put them back, but I had my period.

Fourth attempt I was coming in for my final trial – as usual I was scanned and there it was, this blob in my uterus. I was pregnant and had done it myself!

They sent me off to have my urine tested. I sat there with fingers crossed and I prayed, but I couldn't contain my excitement, I had to tell someone or I would explode with emotion. The other women waiting got involved with the excitement and when the result was positive I hugged the sister and the other women and cried and cried . . . the shock . . . the happiness.

I wanted to call Sunday at work to tell him but I thought this news was too important to tell him over the phone so I asked him to come home early that evening. His response when I told him that I was pregnant was to get angry, 'Emma, how can you joke about such a serious matter.' He couldn't believe that I was pregnant. After all we had been through to have conceived on our own seemed impossible. He waited until the next morning until he called the hospital and heard the news himself before he really believed it and then we celebrated.

EMMA

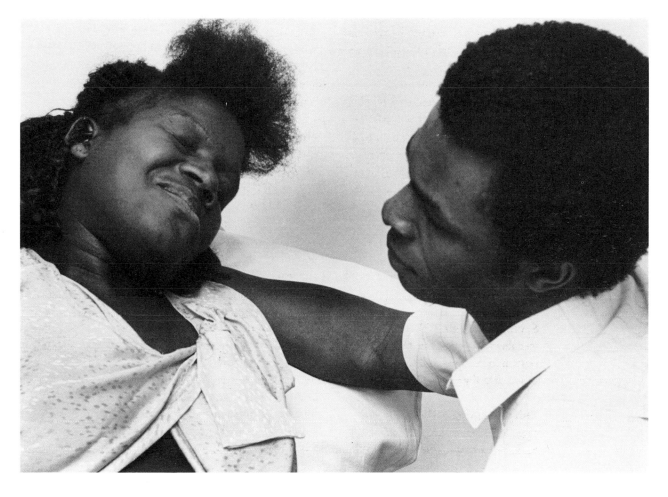

Two weeks before my due date at
5.55am my waters broke with a huge
gush while I was in bed.

I came into the hospital at
7am. I was 3cm dilated. Contractions
were strong and coming every one to
two minutes.

EMMA

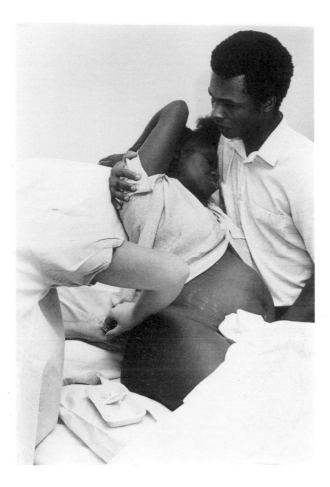

Pethidine was offered for the pain. I declined at first but the contractions were getting much stronger and I was only 3cm dilated. I decided to take it and see how things went.

I felt sick shortly after the 100mg of pethidine was given. The contractions were still painful but possibly less severe than they would have been without the pethidine.

EMMA

I was expecting labour to be painful, I knew that the pain was getting me nearer to the baby, 'nearer to the baby' – the repetition of those words helped me a lot.

The pressure when the baby's head was right down was like a rock a great lump that I had to push out.

EMMA

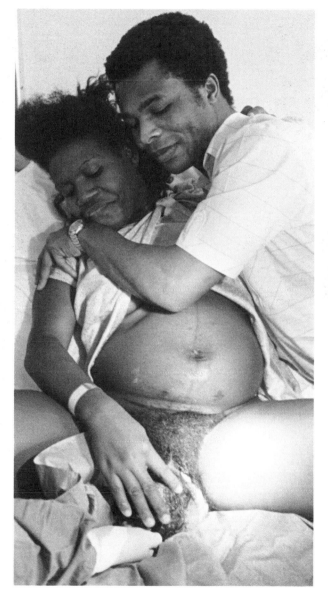

I had feelings of relief and pleasure as I was feeling the baby's head – relief that the pressure was off and pleasure that the baby was here . . . a great, great pleasure. I felt so comfortable at this moment but dreading the next push.

EMMA

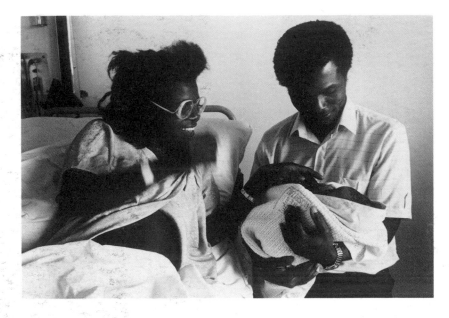

I'll have my sunshine.

EMMA

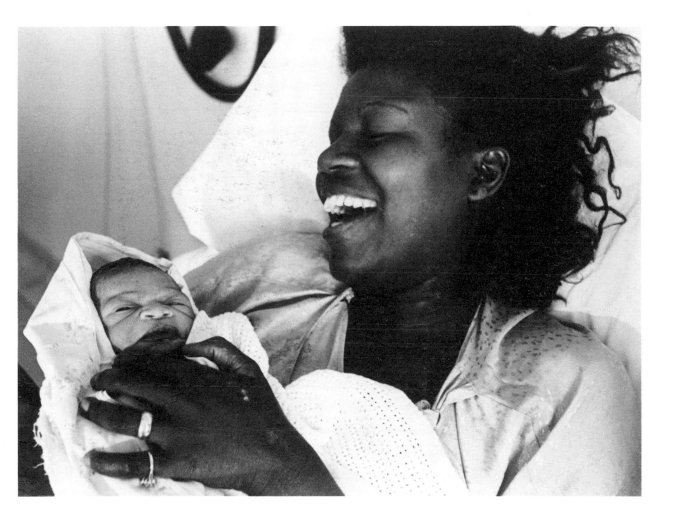

Glossary

Amniocentesis
A test of the amniotic fluid in which the baby floats, carried out at sixteen to eighteen weeks of pregnancy. A needle is inserted through the abdominal wall and uterus to obtain a sample of the fluid which is then tested for a range of congenital abnormalities, including Down's syndrome and spina bifida. Testing varies from hospital to hospital but is generally recommended for women over thirty-seven and those whose families have a history of genetic disorders.

Anterior lip
Part of the cervix. Towards the end of the first stage of labour the anterior lip sometimes remains around the baby's head preventing full dilation of the cervix.

Breech
When a baby is delivered bottom rather than head first.

Epidural
An injection of local anaesthetic into the space around the lower spine which anaesthetises the lower part of the body, from the waist down. Pain relief lasts for about two hours and the anaesthetic can be topped up through a tube which is left in place.

Episiotomy
Cut in the perineum to enlarge the vaginal outlet and help speed delivery.

Gas and air
A mixture of oxygen and nitrous oxide which can be breathed in from a mask before the height of a contraction to help ease the pain of contractions.

Liquor
Alternative term for amniotic fluid, the liquid in which the baby floats in the uterus.

Meconium
A dark, greenish substance; the baby's first bowel movements. If present in the amniotic fluid during labour it may signify that the baby is in distress.

Perineum
The tissue between the vagina and anus.

Pethidine
A narcotic analgesic given by injection during the first stage of labour. It relaxes but its pain relieving effect is variable. It may make the woman feel drowsy and out of control and may also affect the baby.

Syntocinon
A synthetic hormone resembling the natural hormone oxytocin which is produced by the posterior pituitary gland in the brain. Syntocinon is given intravenously to stimulate uterine contractions and thus speed delivery along. It is also usually injected immediately after delivery to help the uterus contract and so facilitate delivery of the placenta.

Vernix
The creamy, water repellant substance which protects the baby's skin when it is born. It comes off gradually after birth.